At the Still Point of the Turning World

T0373010

At the Still Point of the Turning World

The Art and Philosophy of Osteopathy

Robert Lever, DO

Foreword by
R Paul Lee DO, FAAO, FCA

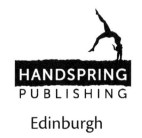

HANDSPRING
PUBLISHING

Edinburgh

HANDSPRING PUBLISHING LIMITED
The Old Manse, Fountainhall,
Pencaitland, East Lothian
EH34 5EY, United Kingdom
Tel: +44 1875 341 859
Website: www.handspringpublishing.com

First published 2013 in the United Kingdom by Handspring Publishing

Copyright ©Handspring Publishing Limited 2013

All rights reserved. No parts of this publication may be reproduced or transmitted in any form
or by any means, electronic or mechanical, including photocopying, recording, or any information storage and retrieval system, without either the prior written permission of the publisher
or a license permitting restricted copying in the United Kingdom issued by the Copyright
Licensing Agency Ltd, Saffron House, 6-10 Kirby Street, London EC1N 8TS.

ISBN 978–1–909141–05–6 Hardback
ISBN 978-1-909141-06-3 Paperback

British Library Cataloguing in Publication Data

A catalogue record for this book is available from the British Library

Design by Pete Wilder, Designers Collective
Artwork by Mark Willey, Designers Collective
Typeset by Palimpsest Book Production Limited
Printed and bound by CPI Group (UK) Ltd, Croydon, CR0 4YY

The
Publisher's
policy is to use
paper manufactured
from sustainable forests

To the memory of

my mentor, Tom Dummer (1915–1998)

and

my father, Derrick Lever (1923–1986)

At the still point of the turning world. Neither flesh nor fleshless;
Neither from nor towards; at the still point, there the dance is,
But neither arrest nor movement. And do not call it fixity,
Where past and future are gathered. Neither movement from nor towards,
Neither ascent nor decline. Except for the point, the still point,
There would be no dance, and there is only the dance.

from 'Burnt Norton', *Four Quartets,* **T.S. Eliot**

Author's note

Writing this book has been both a joy and a challenge, and has, for various reasons had a long incubation period. However, if it had been attempted when it was first mooted (over 25 years ago), it would have been a very different product. One facet of the challenge has been to write about a concept that is in a very real sense 'holographic'. In other words, each part or component of its subject has something to say about every other part and, likewise, is a reflection of them. To put it another way, each ingredient contains something of the whole. This has inevitably meant a degree of repetition as we look at the same thing from different perspectives. It has also meant the necessary fragmentation of a subject that only really 'lives' in its entirety as an integrated whole. As such, the book may read best as a series of essays though there is, I hope, an element of flow and development.

It is my wish that my attempts to express the following ideas, coupled with the reader's willingness to 'join up the dots', will lead to some degree of coherence and a satisfying concoction made from some inspiring ingredients, plucked from a wondrous world itself inspired by osteopathy.

Robert Lever DO

London, March 2013

Contents

Foreword

What is an osteopath? That is the question this book explores. As someone who characterizes himself by that very word, 'osteopath', I have, nevertheless, often wondered what it is that truly defines osteopathy. I have a file in my desk drawer entitled, 'What is a DO?' I have been exploring this question and its companion question, 'What is osteopathy?' since, as a young man, I sold pharmaceuticals to physicians in the USA. When I asked the DOs on my call list these questions, they said the answers were to be found in the education obtained from an osteopathic medical school; and they helped me matriculate at the Kansas City University of Medicine and Biosciences – College of Osteopathic Medicine in 1972. I have been forever grateful.

My gratitude generates from having achieved the understanding, after extensive digging over many years, that osteopathy is as wide and deep as nature herself. Osteopathy is a study and clinical engagement of natural principles. I am occupied on a daily basis in my office as I treat my patients by observing the way nature works. My patients' bodies display fundamental characteristics that reveal, 'How things work.' Dr Still 'discovered' osteopathy, as he said. I believe he did so because he was an ardent observer of nature. He found man to be a machine, the product of spirit, and an example of the perfection of creation. He was interested in the health that is found in the system, the normal that over-rides any dysfunction, as the primary characteristic of the living human. His goal was to use natural principles to re-establish normal structure and function in his patients.

Nature can perform wondrous feats. Look at super storm Sandy or a solar eclipse. When we engage the forces available to us through the sun (solar energy), the moon (tides), the wind and water (stupendous rock formations through erosion), for example, we tap the power of the all-that-is. According to Still, creation emanates from the greater mind, which organizes the material substance and enlivens it with motion – or spirit. He believed that mind, matter, and motion generate all living beings, indeed, the entire universe.

Attending to natural principles, we can listen to the body and discover what it requires to heal. Following its lead, we can assist it in its process, which only the body, itself, can accomplish. We, as osteopaths, support the body in healing itself. We allow the organism to return to its original conformation, which, in turn, allows it to resume its original pace and style of function. In other words, we permit areas of dysfunction within the body to be restored to health. We facilitate the delivery of health to tissues that have been starving for the 'fluids of life,' as Dr Still intimated.

Dr Still indicated that vitalistic principles are responsible for creating the living form, and then, once created, in maintaining its health. Fluids – blood, lymph, and cerebrospinal fluid, as well as other extra-cellular fluids – deliver health. The life force, which creates the living form, also restores the health of the structure by delivering vitalistic principles, as well as nutrients – via fluids. Thus, the rule of the artery is supreme and the CSF is in command, according to William Sutherland, DO. Mechanical (hydraulic) effects characterize the 'potency' of the fluid. Other qualities of potency include electrical potential and the disbursement of information about how the system was created and, as a consequence, how it is to be restored.

Several fellow explorers, including the author of this book, Robert Lever, DO, have rendered untiring pursuit into the meaning of osteopathy. Robert has put together a masterful compilation of essays (chapters), which span the full spectrum of topics from vitality and holism to myth and spirit. In the middle of it all is physics and technique and the questions surrounding placebo and healing. He has taken the discussion about osteopathy to a new level, redefining the profession in terms that are modern and far seeing. If anyone has followed Dr Still's admonition to 'Dig On,' it is Robert Lever, with this excellent effort.

One must read what he has to say and work outward – from all the details to the whole of it – to perceive what he wants us to understand. Although entertaining, intriguing and very informative, this book is not a simple read-through. It is necessary to study what he declares: 'It is the fortunate interplay of the body's systems in a complex web of interaction that allows the osteopath . . . to access the potential that draws on the powerful process of self-correction.' Then, we can find the larger meaning: 'The resilience, adaptability and capacity for survival in human beings are, at times as extraordinary as they are mysterious.'

When it comes to defining or, for that matter, practising osteopathy, we can find many opinions and styles. This volume, *At The Still Point of the Turning World* views differing opinions from the author's British perspective. Although the issues might vary slightly due to a century of separate development of the British and American versions of osteopathy, in the USA, we are no different. We hold many opinions and sometimes they can lead to disagreement. Robert Lever has attempted to unify our variations on a theme by tracing the differences to their origin and then melding them under simpler principles. This is a valuable effort by him. Its success depends upon individual osteopaths being as willing to trace, as well and thoroughly as the author, these fundamentals that he cites. Its success also depends upon the reader being as willing as the author to look at the larger picture and to accept a worldview that might be different from what he/she first believed.

Dr Still held a worldview that was contrary to the majority of the people of his day. Despite being rejected from all quarters – his family, friends, colleagues, as well as the clergy – he persisted, because he knew he was following the truth where it led him in his quest. Today, it is no different. If we are to fulfill the potential of osteopathy, as huge as it is – as big as all of nature – we must be willing to look at it through new spectacles. We must follow Dr Still's command, 'Dig On!' Robert Lever's effort, in this volume, is a wonderful step in that direction. I applaud him for his insight that derives from a life of osteopathic clinical experience, teaching and contemplation. Indeed, Robert Lever is a teacher to us all.

R. Paul Lee, DO, FAAO, FCA
Durango, Colorado, USA
January 2013

Preface

Some years ago, when I was a first-year student, a delightful lecturer would speak in amusing terms about all sorts of bodily functions as a light-hearted introduction to physiology. Lecturers then – as now – often held one's attention through style and delivery rather than content! However, he memorably spoke about practice life as series of situations in which one would need to cultivate an interest in anything and everything the patient might wish to share. An early lesson in empathy, he would say with characteristic mimes and hand movements to embellish his point: you'll need to be fascinated by golf, train-spotting, bricklaying . . . anything. And whereas I could well imagine finding patients' enthusiasms infectious, I was sure the line would have to be drawn, for me anyway, at hunting and philately.

Some time later, a patient *did* want to share his passion for philately and sure enough, the seduction began as he described stamps as little windows on history and, once again, I was 'hooked', all was well. I'm not sure in all my years of practice that I have yet been tested with bricklaying but I suppose I'm open to it should the need arise.

About 40-odd years ago, as part of my passion for virtuoso piano music, I listened to an interview with the great Vladimir Horowitz. Music and the piano have remained an obsession for me. At the time, Horowitz said that in order to be a fine pianist, the artist had to interest himself in many things apart from music. I don't think he had bricklaying or philately in mind but he did refer to painting, theatre, dance, history and the arts in general.

Two things emerge from this preamble. The first is that one can often be drawn into an appreciation of a subject unexpectedly, to find a richness in it that one might otherwise judge simplistically, ignore, or even, by virtue of misunderstanding or misinterpretation, completely reject. The other is that any field of interest can be enriched by incorporating or including seemingly unrelated material which can educate and broaden it in remarkable ways, ways that may not only be important but vital to the pursuit of excellence in that field. In my view, both of these apply to osteopathy and though this is not a textbook about osteopathy, it's where it all starts for me. To put it simply, theory and practice are immeasurably enhanced by breadth of interest and breadth of understanding. Meanwhile, it is my contention that the practice of osteopathy has struggled in two major respects. The first is an incomplete grasp and implementation of the principle of Holism; and the second is the somewhat awkward incorporation of what I call the 'subjective' element in practice, to balance and refine its theoretical basis. My intention is to elaborate both these themes throughout this book and to suggest the importance of wider aspects of humanity to the art of osteopathic practice.

SPACES AND GLUE

Whether we look at concepts, ideas or even objects themselves, it is the 'spaces' between them, their juxtaposition or 'interface', their interaction, that 'contain' properties that whilst hard to define, produce the glue that gives things complexity, depth and meaning. There are many things in life whose value is to be found in 'the glue', the interface. If we fail to look there and appreciate 'wholes' instead of 'parts', we are left with ideas, concepts, theories or statements that are limited, meaningless or simply wrong. Many areas of human endeavour have been rejected or ignored through such a failure of observation so that things of inestimable value have been consigned to the scrap-heap of vilified unorthodoxy. Very often, these brave efforts have been spawned by cultures, traditions and folklore, although sometimes they can emerge as 'new' paradigms such as systems theory, holism and some of the revelations spawned by quantum theory. We'll consider the impact of these on our particular field later in the chapters that follow.

Osteopathy has been my profession, my working obsession, for about 40 years. It has been augmented, informed and elaborated by many things 'non-osteopathic' and 'non-medical', with every day's experience. It has also been a window on a wider world of understanding and exploration that has produced many philosophical meanderings, spiritual reflections and much questioning. Many a time have my former students' eyes glazed over as I launched into more of these forays when I knew their minds were troubled by more pressing matters: the next day's neurology exam or whatever. However, two or three used to like to join me for the ride, and that sharing could create some of the most enjoyable moments of my teaching experience. Some have claimed since that I articulated things that they've been keen to crystallise, explore or clarify so I feel some justification in continuing the sharing through this book.

A great deal of what I'll express in these pages is a reflection of my own personal perspective, process and experience. I can't really claim any startling originality, after all, it is often said that everything has already been said before; we merely find new clothes for old ideas. Even so, now and then, radically new perspectives are born that are the product of truly creative minds. This piece of work belongs, if it belongs anywhere, in the former category, the 'new clothes' department! Be that as it may, I've long been grateful for what I can only describe as my good fortune to enjoy just how much my practice as an osteopath has taught and revealed to me. And having revelled in some of the many 'interfaces' that have presented themselves, I've wanted not only to express the way that the art of osteopathy transcends its vital scientific underpinnings, but also celebrate aspects of what makes us human, as well as layers of interest that can be made available to the open, hungry and surrendering mind through this work.

Many of these journeys lead to strange regions, intellectual abstractions, philosophical tangles, questions without answers of course, and spiritual forays that engender a sense of wonder and mystery, part of the 'food' of life and thought (for some, anyway). Above all, I've wanted to find an alternative to the suffocating tendency of our times to grant validity only to those practices that are reducible to proven facts. By eliminating the world of the 'subjective', we cut that world in half.

However, I've also wanted to look at the places where science has attempted to break away from the mainstream, just as osteopathy itself broke away from medicine in the 1870s. This is often the exciting world of the mavericks who push boundaries through the sheer power, determination and inspiration of their exploring minds, and I've wanted to celebrate the way these serious-minded explorations have lent our osteopathic discipline clarity to illuminate much of what we've done well without always knowing why. As Karen Armstrong states with reference to the belated evidence for Einstein's theory of relativity: 'In science, as in theology, human beings could make progress on unproven ideas, which worked practically even if they had not [yet] been demonstrated empirically' (Armstrong, 2009).

Osteopaths will, I hope, find an interest in some of this. Much of it they will know or take issue with, for it is well known that osteopaths rarely agree about anything! (Indeed, there will be some detractors who take a very different view of our work, having little time for some of the ideas expressed in this book.) But non-osteopaths might find something in it too whether or not they have had any connection with osteopathy as patients or professionals of other persuasions. For in the end, I feel our searching in life is always about more than any one circumscribed area of enquiry, whether it be within a professional discipline, a career, a hobby, even a spiritual or religious calling.

The art of osteopathy – not just its concepts, theories or techniques – is one of many pathways studded with signs, illuminations, insights and tantalising blind alleys that often point towards something greater and more mysterious than we can ever know but which as human beings we will never be able to resist. And though there are many such ways, the art of osteopathy is one way of working with what makes us 'human'. It just happens that osteopathy has been my particular path.

What makes osteopathy live is based on what 'informs' it. Once alive, it illuminates so much in the human domain. It's my wish to share some of that rather than produce a textbook or manual. Also, in this regard, I've wanted to counter the somewhat 'binary', tick-box, target-oriented approach to everything that increasingly permeates the healthcare professions (and most other professions too), even when holistic pretentions are claimed; 'respectability' and conformity have been bought and the price has been 'fragmentation'.

Like most things in life, osteopathic practice at its best is a 'seamless whole', an integrated experience, and to break it down into parts is to risk distortion. However, in order to communicate its qualities, it has been necessary to indulge in a certain amount of 'analysis'. Such analysis, even though subjected to the principles of 'holism' and the notion of interconnectedness, can have a tendency to fragment truths and experience, creating a note of 'separateness' or specialisation alongside that 'interconnectedness'. My intention is that the reader might ultimately find this book helpful in joining the dots up again in a useful and meaningful way, whereby we can come to see mind *in* body, body *in* mind and spirit in both.

It could be said that osteopathy only really exists as it's being 'performed'. It is an abstraction until it takes root in our humanity or the humanity of its exponents. Like music, it may be based on theory, technique and 'context', but at some point, interpretation has to be transformed into something greater, whether to produce the music that speaks to us or treatment that penetrates and heals. In our work at its best, each practitioner brings something unique to the practice that expresses something quite individual. This, as I shall argue, is its strength. Therefore, I've been at pains to explore some of the qualities that make us who and what we are. Perhaps because of this, the book has been written from a somewhat personal perspective. Meanwhile I trust that there are enough resonances for others to make it more than a self-indulgent exercise!

Readers will, perhaps, have varying levels of interest in the subject, depending whether inside or outside the profession. Those outside might prefer to glide superficially over the more technical bits, though I've been at pains not to make it overly technical. Hopefully the rest will make up for it.

SCIENCE VS SPIRIT

In the later chapters in particular, some might think that this book places itself at the centre of an argument between science and 'spirit'. But this is not intended. If anything, it reflects on the schism between 'scientism' and philosophy (pure science and philosophy having formerly been more comfortably entwined) or between what we often try, with closed minds, to assert as *fact* on the one hand, and those profound speculations born of man's journeys in to the 'unknown' on the other, the latter being common to both 'good' science *and* philosophy. If there *is* a dichotomy, it is between the 'known' and the 'unknown'. One of the messages in this book is that, for the art of osteopathy to thrive, they both matter—in equal degrees but in different ways.

Many will know that science and scientists place themselves at the threshold of this *unknown*; this is, after all, their job. And as such, theirs are amongst the most creative of minds. The problems lie more with the *culture* of science (*scientism*) and the limitations sometimes imposed by closed minds in which value is ascribed only to that which is already proven. The art of healing has been threatened with emasculation by the rigid application of this idea. However, the picture is changing owing to profound changes in science itself, a 'paradigm shift' so enormous that its assimilation into mainstream thinking, medical and otherwise, is taking time. It is, after all, a messy process: Arthur Koestler wrote that revolutions in science and knowledge emerge out of the chaos created when paradigms break down (Peat, 1989). Such chaos causes much insecurity which, in turn, produces some very negative and destructive argument; these positions have done very little to illuminate much wisdom or truth. And whereas empiricism has become a benchmark for the scientific method, it was, from Aristotle onwards, linked to knowledge based on the experience *via the senses*; the blending of both objective and subjective faculties.

As regards the 'spirit/science' dichotomy (for those who insist there is one), if it has any relevance at all, it is in the pursuit of understanding about 'reality' in the external world. The *inner* world at its most profound is one of subjective experience and here, scientific analysis can only help us so far (if at all). After all, by and large, people are not driven by the need to know the nature of 'reality'; their lives are generated by other impulses. And as Wittgenstein stated: '*we feel that even when all possible scientific questions have been answered, the problems of life remain completely untouched*' (Wittgenstein, 1921).

In his book *Body Myths,* medical anthropologist, Cecil Helman (1991), wrote: 'In all societies, people live their lives in a sea of metaphor and myth, gathered together from many sources.'

Ananda Coomaraswamy (1943) had previously stated that 'myth embodies the nearest approach to absolute truth that can be stated in words.' The 'creation' of osteopathy involved the distillation of some great truths. However, as I'll suggest several times, most if not all truths defy complete analysis, description and language. Words distort by de-contextualising ideas. Perhaps that's why Einstein once said, 'I often think in music.' But as I don't aspire to such genius and as I can't paint, write poetry or compose string quartets, this piece of work will have to do.

London, March 2013   **Robert Lever DO**

REFERENCES:

Armstrong, K, 2009, *The Case for God,* The Bodley Head, 256–7.
Coomaraswamy, A K, 1943, *Hinduism and Buddhism,* Philosophical Library, New York.
Helman, C, 1991, *Body Myths,* Chatto & Windus.
Peat, F D, Dec 1989, *Edges Magazine.*
Wittgenstein, L, 1921, *Tractus Logico-Philosophicus,* Routledge.

Part 1

Principles

Chapter 1

Osteopathy: an overview

Healing, Papa would tell me, *is not a science, but the intuitive art of wooing Nature.*

(W H Auden: *The Art of Healing*)

In our professional role, we as osteopaths spend a lot of time helping patients find answers: 'answers' to help with pain and other symptoms, ailments or complaints. Sometimes this is purely palliative, sometimes part of a quest for better health. Sometimes it's a way of addressing deeper struggles or attempts to find meaning and reasons for things. This may help patients find ways of controlling their problems, if not their destiny! Meanwhile, the search for meaning and control is, perhaps, the driving force behind most if not all of our endeavours in the context of what it is to be human, but the drive towards 'structural balance and integrity' and everything that this enables, is what dominates osteopathic thinking. And what is truly remarkable is just what this *does* enable and the potential for change that it can afford on so many levels of human function and experience. I sincerely hope that this book goes some way towards showing why this is possible, why it happens in daily practice, and something of the process by which we can help it to make it happen.

Background

Osteopathy, or osteopathic medicine as it is sometimes called, is one of many windows on the wider world of meaning whether its purpose is focused on the relief of pain, a pathway to improved health, a means of coping or finding a sense of direction or purpose, that precious quest without end, or simply on helping people live more comfortably 'inside their own skins.' And as such, osteopathy is one form of 'interpretation', one of many approaches that dedicates itself to making things better. However, it has managed to acquire a number of stereotypical misconceptions over the years about what it is and what it purports to do and when it 'states' its potential honestly, it is often viewed as pretentious, over-ambitious or even arrogant. One of the reasons for this is that its methods and its theoretical basis are viewed against the backdrop of a highly developed medical sophistication and technology that are of a very different cultural flavour. Osteopathy and mainstream medicine may well have approximately similar goals – healing – but they are conceptually as different as painting and music. When osteopathy was conceived, it was both a reaction, almost a revolution, and an alternative. But above all, it was a new way of seeing; a way of conceptualising health and disease that called for a new way of treating patients. Indeed, its methods were dedicated to the 'location', enhancement and expression of *health* in the patient more than the confrontation of disease *per se.*

Misconceptions

Let's look at misconceptions about osteopathy first and then at its evolution over its 150 years' history. Sit next to a perfect stranger at that sometimes grim phenomenon known as the dinner party and naturally enough and pretty soon the subject of one's occupation will arise. All of us in the profession will have heard one of the stock responses: 'what's that?' (although this is becoming rarer in the last 30 years); or 'oh that's bones isn't it?'; or, 'oh that's backs'; or the 'tabloid-oriented' might gleefully recall Stephen Ward – 'society osteopath'– and the notorious 'Profumo scandal' of the 1960s, imagining us to have equally colourful if not scandalous lives; or perhaps someone will launch into a description of back-related pain that invites on-the-spot consultation. One colleague would circumvent the tedium of such conversations, bringing them to an abrupt close with the words, 'Actually, I sell spoons'! Well, given that things like that don't happen without a reason, why is it that members of the public have so little idea about osteopathic medicine unless, that is, they have personally experienced osteopathy at its broadest and best? Why has Andrew Taylor Still's vision been so poorly understood and interpreted?

The question is really a far deeper one and not only involves the problem that any society or culture has with the integration of new ideas but also the resistance to embrace new perspectives. When Dr Still established osteopathy in the 1870s, he was already a practising physician and for reasons known to many in the profession (see below), he propounded the concept of osteopathy as an *alternative,* not as an extension of conventional medical practice. Now as much as we need and teach medical science in its conventional guise and integrate it into the whole matter of patient care, the true practice of osteopathy has to sidestep conventional methods, *almost* completely, to base its diagnostic and therapeutic practice on a very different paradigm.

It has been said that if a new idea involves too many logical steps to integrate it into the established canon of knowledge, it will remain on the sidelines where it will be consigned to 'cranky' unorthodoxy at best and oblivion at worst. Alfred Pischinger (1899–1982), for example, who pioneered research into the significance of the extracellular matrix and its role in disease causation made such a valuable contribution to a truer understanding of disease, yet his work was too radical to be absorbed into the mainstream and has been largely ignored or forgotten. Comparatively recently it has been resuscitated as its relevance is being realized, more particularly within those disciplines that focus on the *predisposition* to disease rather than the confrontation of it. But we'll look at this more a little later.

Meanwhile, the culture of scepticism daily rejects so-called 'alternative' approaches, blind to their complexity, seeing them as transgressions of what is anyway an incomplete and sometimes erroneous 'orthodox' medical concept whose adherents remain convinced of its infallibility. Add to this the weight of the establishment/mainstream credo, and the integration of alternative principles can become a forlorn hope with as much promise of meaningful dialogue as an acrimonious divorce. I often think that the articulate and intelligent critics of alternative methods might sometimes temper their certainty with a willingness to look outside their beautifully crafted conceptual boxes. To be genuinely and constructively discriminating is to 'let go' of certainty, to allow knowledge to point the way *towards* the unknown, rather than merely to underscore the already proven.

PARADIGMS

In his classic text *The Structure of Scientific Revolutions* (1962) on the crisis essential to the 'paradigm shift', a phrase he coined, Thomas Kuhn elucidates for all time the way that major advances in science and knowledge 'happen' rather than 'evolve'. The happening may well require an evolution of thought but it is when the creative leap occurs that innovation is truly born. This might be the result of inspiration, intuition, divine intervention or sheer genius or the overlapping of all these, but it *occurs* rather than develops, often as a by-product of the methodical search for something else. What is virtually inevitable is the way that innovation is resisted, feared and rejected, though what I'm afraid sometimes 'oils the wheels' of acceptance, might be political or commercial expediency. (Clearly, in this respect, no one had much to gain from the integration of osteopathy into health care, at least not for a while!)

What is worse for osteopathy is that as a profession, it has reacted to ostracism by bargaining with the establishment and attempting to dress itself in 'respectable' clothes, even believing that it should conform to the conventional model to gain acceptance. Sadly, this has created a schism in the profession but more strangely, it has as a trend ignored the fact that medical science is itself changing all the time while some in our own profession cling to worn-out models! Some of the newer models have evolved from contemporary physics and this has provided some of the most exciting underpinnings of the osteopathic method that we have known. The problem is that these innovations in science are truly challenging and their proponents have similar problems of acceptance amongst many of their peers. But here, it has to be said and said loudly, that if 'new' knowledge simply exaggerated and elaborated what we knew already, nothing much would have changed in the history of civilisation.

Likewise, if musicians and artists had never offended established opinions and tastes (which many of the great ones did), their art would have died from stultification. Allowing for the vagaries of fashion, many have broken new ground to drive their art forward, celebration only gradually replacing vilification and derision. Look, for example, at the public reaction to Manet, Turner, Van Gogh, Scriabin and Stravinsky. Time would have to pass before their influence and pivotal place in the evolution of their artistic fields would be appreciated, respected and acclaimed. The breaking of new ground, so vital for progress, inevitably entails the radical restructuring of the 'established', whose minions and devotees are profoundly threatened and outraged by change.

I am not too concerned here with writing a history of osteopathy; others have tackled this task admirably, many within the profession will be fairly familiar with it and others of my readers might have only marginal interest in it. However there are certain aspects that seem to engage people. One is the misconception that osteopathy is derived from eastern culture; a view that many of our patients have voiced. Many eastern philosophical and spiritual ideas have certainly influenced some aspects of practice for several – though certainly not all – practitioners. However, osteopathy was born in the United States, in Missouri; delivered into the world by a physician, Andrew Taylor Still, who was born in Virginia and whose father was a Methodist minister in a predominantly farming community. Various cultural influences might well have shaped Still's ideas since his time living and working with the Shwanee Indians in the 1850s, but osteopathy was an American import.

STILL AND ORIGINS

There can be very little doubt that Dr Still saw his version of medicine as a radical alternative to the medicine of the day. Many patients and their families come to us now for the same reason, as an alternative to the mainstream. Still's reasons were very personal. He had lost three children from spinal meningitis and this experience filtered through his almost obsessive musings on the body, on what we would now call functional anatomy, and on the natural order of things. Still was a highly spiritual man though he probably had little time for formal religion, and his spiritual sense expanded his philosophical approach to the human condition that led to the assertion of a *vitalistic* principle that expressed the potential for health and repair in the body, provided that certain conditions were met, a dynamic propensity that he called 'biogen'. This potential was based on the principle of unity of function (integration), the biochemical mechanism of self-regulation, and the prime requisite of healthy physical and mechanical 'adjustment'. The idea that the balanced complex integration of the body structure – most importantly including the fascia – being intimately related to health, healing and self-repair was born. So was an approach to manual treatment that was designed to enhance it, and Still called it 'osteopathy'.

Now, however complex the art of this work may be and however hard it is to acquire the necessary skills of diagnosis, palpation and technique, this notion can sometimes appear banal in the face of the medical sophistication that we are so used to in the orthodox arena. But it was ever thus. Still's ideas were ground-breaking, and although he had derived some of his ideas from pioneers in other fields, it was his inspiration to bring them together in the form of a medical discipline or system, to advocate an almost passionate interest in anatomy and to assert the relationship between 'structure' and 'function' that was to form the basis for the system that has been practised for 150 years. The orthodoxy of Still's time simply couldn't wear it and frankly, many would say they haven't really worn it since! However, we're still here and though many in the profession have felt the squeeze of disapproval from the medical establishment and have sought a more comfortable place within it, involving a significant compromise of principle, there are others who see Still's truths as vividly as ever, whose practice is based on them and who continue to explore available developments in science that validate the work and Still's gift.

Some inside the profession will be disappointed by my reluctance to have osteopathy conform theoretically or methodologically to conventional medical discipline. Such conformity – for either politically expedient reasons or through the bowing under the weight of medicine's undisputed achievements – would be disingenuous. Osteopathy has always been a different discipline with strengths that are its *raisons d'être*. Without them, and by compromising to become an 'add-on' to the structural end of medicine, we would gradually lose our role and cease to be, with our unique voice. Some would say such a danger is closer than we think. Furthermore, the ambiguous relationship between osteopathy and the mainstream has taken many different forms in different parts of the world. In some countries, it is illegal; in others it is permitted but only if practised by medical doctors; in many, it exists as an independently regulated profession, as in the UK; and somewhat paradoxically, in the USA, the birthplace of osteopathy, it has undergone a political 'mutation', in which it has donned the guise, training and discipline of the allopathic profession leaving a tiny minority who have continued 'on the path'.

When Theresa Cisler edited and produced the compilation of impassioned writings of one of osteopathy's elder statesmen, Bob Fulford, under the title *Are We On The Path?* (2003), it posed the very real challenge to the profession that, in many respects, we weren't. The struggle that the profession has experienced with this 'true' relationship with our principles may have been partly conceptual and intellectual but it has also been largely political and expedient, and this has, as I say, played out differently in different countries and at different times.

Still's language, his almost poetic turns of phrase, the relatively unsophisticated levels of medical understanding of his time compared with our own, all these make Still hard, even for some of our own number, to take. But in common with so many innovative ideas, so many inspirational truths, language reveals its shortcomings. So often in what we now call 'holistic' thinking, we deal with such an infinite sense of *unity or oneness* as a concept that we truly run out of language, reaching out for metaphor. We need to read Still with this in mind, and this applies too when we look at the work of our other early pioneers like William Garner Sutherland who we'll meet in Chapter 5.

But here, I must highlight a common tendency: an arrogance of attitude that often consigns historical material to inferior, even doubtful status at best, to the scrap heap at worst. Instead of seeing new material as a product of a different perspective, we see it as something that supersedes everything that went before. Now, whereas this is, of course, sometimes true, it isn't always the case. There has been a tendency in our profession to reject some of our finer concepts in the name of 'progress' in order to conform within a paradigm that best fits another discipline all together.

DIVERSITY

Many different styles and perspectives pepper the profession of osteopathy. As I frequently tell patients: osteopathy is not a standard product. The same can of course be said about all medical disciplines, both conventional and otherwise. Surgeons will differ in the way they perform certain operations and will bring varying levels of skill to their task. I often say to students, ponder the difference between a competent surgeon and a great one. The skills involved are a product to some extent of dexterity, but the experiential and technical knowledge brought to bear, the intuitive sense of 'feel' derived from years of experience, wise clinical judgement, the empathy and involvement with the tissues and their anatomy, all these contribute to a performance of real distinction and excellence. The same is certainly true of osteopathy (as well as many other therapeutic skills). Training, clinical perspectives, inspiration, personality all combine with competence to provide a 'product' that is in some ways unique, and our role as teachers should, to some extent, be directed at helping our students make the art 'their own.'

Good teaching sows the seeds of these skills. It is their germination that not only supports the growth of the individual student's special abilities, but in harnessing these to principles of diagnosis and treatment that have been tried and tested over many years, it furnishes the student with the potential to develop as a clinician that should always keep the work fresh, open to new perspectives and alive. For, in the end, there are no definitive treatments. We prime the student with principle and method and then encourage the individual to fashion the rest through a process of dedication.

Learning, styles and schools

On the odd occasion that patients have been impressed with proceedings during a treatment, they've asked: how do you learn how to do this? How do you teach it? This always reminds me of my opening remarks with every new cohort of students when I say, much to their chagrin, I can't teach you how to *do* osteopathy – sad because that's usually why they're there – but what I will try to do is plant enough seeds of thought and orientation that the skills, attitudes and 'approach' will begin to develop in you such that you can begin to make the craft 'your own', grafting it on to the applied scientific foundations and techniques of osteopathic medicine. The more mature and patient ones can accept this; others fume with frustration.

However, the succinct if somewhat simplified response to the patient might sum up the bare bones of it and I'll say:

- We teach the student about 'structure' (anatomy)
- We teach the student about 'function' (physiology)
- We teach them how these relate to one another
- We teach them about normal function of the parts
- We teach them about abnormal function (pathology)
- We help them to recognise *abnormal* function of parts; relationships and malrelationships
- We show them how this is relevant to the clinical picture or presentation – osteopathically
- We teach methods of correction; technique, treatment methods and approaches
- We teach them *when* to rectify/correct, i.e. strategy
- And (traditionally and ideally) we steep it all in a firm and emphatic grounding in osteopathic principles and clinical medicine.

But I then explain that there are many styles and perspectives when it comes to the implementation of these basic ideas, and the teaching of them is subject to often wide variations. However, the refining of the necessary skills involves a curious process that is perhaps common to several holistic disciplines and that could roughly be expressed in terms of 'questions we ask the body', in our case, through informed palpation and observation. The strands of information that we seek are intertwined and are broadly described in the list of 'structure/function bonds' below. However, we develop our skills in an almost organic way:

- We acquire the ability to observe more and more strands of information while understanding more and more about their interaction or mutual influence. In this way, we develop the facility to see what the answer to each 'question' contributes to all other answers. The answers themselves relate to the patient's clinical, personal and life issues that are reflected in the body and its tissue responses that we interpret to create a diagnostic 'pattern'; a pattern that is formed via the implementation of a model that, for us, is based in 'structure'. The model itself incorporates the 'structure/function bonds' to which I've referred.

The reason students get better at this is because they become more receptive to more informational 'strands' contained in the presenting case and to recognise their potential interconnections with more rapidity and interpretative skill. This is why palpation improves. One acquires the facility to attend to one issue whilst being open to many others and to understand their relevance to one another. Each palpated structure contains functional relevance or significance, particularly in its relationship to its structural and functional contexts. This way, palpation reveals more.

So when a structure is palpated, it is necessary to understand its significance, anatomically, physiologically and 'reciprocally', with its potential for almost limitless interaction with the rest of the body, all in the same moment. One interprets structure through an appreciation of its total significance and role. In other words, palpation of a structure is to become informed about its functional significance in relation to other structures, as well as neurophysiological and circulatory dynamics, emotional and 'energetic' expression (perhaps), and subtle informational exchange through the connective tissue matrix of the entire body. In the light of this, many would say that diagnosis is 90% of the task.

STYLES

So, back to styles and perspectives. My experience and focus are largely centred on osteopathy in the UK and so it is here that I place my emphasis. Osteopathy here as elsewhere is an expression of its schools, its teachers and the odd 'guru' whose followers sometimes assert their chosen methods with an almost religious fervour. The claims to the only 'real' osteopathic truth have often created division in the profession and it took many years before the profession in this country would find some measure of unity and begin to speak with something resembling one voice. When it did, it did so for largely political reasons and it was correct to do so, for it had struggled with the lack of acceptance and with political and professional ostracism for many years, partly due to the failure to define itself through any kind of unity of thought. But having said that, diversity can spawn richness and depth and where differences can be celebrated, the scope for growth and greater understanding is always enhanced. Meanwhile the distinctions that are often drawn between these diverse approaches remain fundamental differences in style and application rather than principle, and it is my view that any assertion to the contrary is based on misinterpretation. To explore the overlap here is fruitful and revealing; to languish in the realm of 'mutual exclusivity' is not, and has split the profession many times in its history. Differing styles and approaches within osteopathy (with their respective emphasis on 'structure', 'fluids' and 'energetics', 'voluntary' versus 'involuntary' mechanisms etc.) all share a resonance with one another through an adherence to basic principle; they not only aim to arrive 'at the same place' (patient benefit etc.); at their best, they also *derive* from the same place: the conceptual framework that osteopathy has always been which is present at the root of all these approaches when properly interpreted.

SCHOOLS

As I've said, osteopathy was an American import and it became rooted in the UK very largely due to the contribution of John Martin Littlejohn (1865–1947) and the establishing of the British School of Osteopathy in 1915 (receiving its charter in 1917). Although osteopathy had 'appeared' in this country prior to Littlejohn's return from the USA in 1913, largely through some of the early graduates of the first American schools and the creation of the British Osteopathic Association in 1911, it was to be Littlejohn's contribution to osteopathy and osteopathic education that was to establish osteopathy in this country. The teaching of osteopathy was not confined to the BSO in these early years. The Northern Counties School was established in 1925 and the Looker School in 1920, the latter formerly known as the Manchester School that had trained such luminaries as Willis Haycock who contributed so much to the understanding of 'functional technique' in the UK. After Littlejohn's death in 1947, the direction of the British School of Osteopathy (BSO) was the product of the contributions of Stanley Webster-Jones, Clem Middleton, Margot Gore and Audrey Smith (Lady Percival). Soon after, Colin Dove was to enter the fray with his lasting contribution to osteopathic education and osteopathic politics, and there have been four principals since, with Martin Collins in post from 1998 to the present day.

Osteopathic education in the UK was, for many years dominated by the British School of Osteopathy, The British College of Naturopathy & Osteopathy – now The British College of Osteopathic Medicine (BCOM), and The European School of Osteopathy (ESO). Now, there are eight other training establishments in the UK (including the London School of Osteopathy and The College of Osteopaths, and the postgraduate course for doctors at the London College of Osteopathic Medicine established in 1946), that are also recognised by the General Osteopathic Council, but for many years, these three schools, the BSO, ESO and BCOM, produced the bulk of graduates in this country and they created their own 'celebrities', nuances, styles and followings.

BCOM was originally established in 1936 and its training was a hybrid that was based on Naturopathic principles into which osteopathy was woven (or more accurately, appended). The guiding force behind the naturopathic ethos was Stanley Lief who had a pioneering role in the Nature Cure movement in the UK. The osteopathic ingredient in the course had many different flavours depending on the composition of the faculty of the time and ranged from a sort of 'manipulative adjunct 'attached to the naturopathic core of dietetic, hydrotherapeutic and 'lifestyle' prescriptions, through to a keener and truer osteopathic teaching under those such as John Wernham, Thomas Dummer and others. When these two (along with three or four other members of faculty) 'broke away' from the college to expand the Ecole Française d'Ostéopathie, later the Ecole Européene d'Ostéopathie (the tutorial course established by Paul Geny in 1951 and partly run in London for European students) and to create the ESO in 1974 under the stewardship of Tom Dummer as principal, it was largely to dedicate itself to a broad spectrum of teaching with a true and profound emphasis on osteopathic principles. Interestingly, these two men (Dummer and Wernham) represented and taught two almost polarised styles of osteopathy, but for some years, were happy to celebrate (later 'tolerate') their differences as representative of two perspectives on the same theme. (Later, they parted company and Wernham retreated to his long- established Institute of Applied Technique to create the Maidstone College of Osteopathy which since 1996 has continued as The John Wernham College of Classical Osteopathy). This diversity was expanded hugely and energetically when the ESO 'imported' other flavours too, including such approaches as 'cranial' osteopathy, 'functional technique', 'muscle energy technique', 'strain and counterstrain', BLT or 'balanced ligamentous tension' and others, and to knit them, for the first time, into undergraduate training. This involved the developing of fraternal relationships with many of the experts in these fields, (several from the USA, including Bill Johnston, McFarlane Tilley, Larry Jones, John Upledger, Fred Mitchell and many others), so that these special skills could be introduced with authenticity. It was Dummer's extraordinary ability to embrace this diversity and to harness it under one roof that gave the ESO its remarkable quality and produced an almost meteoric rise in popularity, the demand for its course growing rapidly in both the UK and internationally. While this eclecticism posed real challenges to the students, its benefits in providing breadth and depth of osteopathic understanding was considerable.

Meanwhile, what I'd like to emphasise is that although these and other schools created their own flavours based on their own traditions, the thread of osteopathy was common to them all. However, that thread has held such elusive truths that it has at times suffered the potential for profound misunderstanding and misinterpretation, and the schools have all struggled in their own ways to forge a relationship with the principles of osteopathy, resulting in much intellectual and philosophical argument. The struggle to thoroughly assimilate osteopathic wisdom has not only been amongst the orthodox medical sphere. Many within the profession have been tempted to pare it down to a more 'palatable', less elusive product that has been at serious risk of degenerating into a rather dull form of 'manipulative medicine' that lacks depth, penetration and the facility to work broadly with human ills or more correctly, with human health, in the way that our heritage revealed to us.

How does it all work?

The process by which osteopathy *can* access human health and in so doing assist in the process of resolution is profound and complex. It is not an anti-dotal system of health care that has a remedy for every ailment. But all too often, detractors within the profession have sought to have osteopathy conform to this 'tick-box' approach and to sacrifice the art, power and potency of this healing craft, all in the interests of modernity, bringing osteopathy 'up to date' and eliminating all that 'quaint' rather archaic stuff! Sadly, almost tragically, the profession faces that same schism today.

Fortunately, however, there are several within all the schools, their faculties, and their hundreds of graduates, who are 'digging deeper' as Still entreated, who are inspired by the vibrant message of osteopathy and who wish passion-ately to keep it alive. The cultural tide and its materialistic flavour make it rather hard-going but firstly, its truths are worth preserving. Secondly, if we are diligent in the way we explore and draw on cutting-edge science, we will continue to substantiate and validate these truths and the inspiration of our pioneers. The task isn't easy, not least because the cutting-edge science itself, like all radical moves forward, is meeting its own resistance within its own academic fields.

So, next and for those unacquainted with them, let's look at just how the innovative ideas of 'structure/function' interdependency have appeared and manifested in the osteopathic mind over the ages and these extraordinary ingredients of which I, along with many others, am so protective.

Many of them are, of course, second nature to the vast majority of our students. Some of them are not and some of these are amongst the most exciting and the most significant. But just what is it that underpins the concept of osteopathic practice? Later chapters will explore some of this in the sense of what brings it all alive, makes it live and makes it relevant to human beings and their bodies. But for now, let's look at the basic tenets and discuss the way that ideas have broadened over the years.

Structure/function

Firstly, what does this 'structure/function' principle really mean?

It means that the health and mechanical integration of the body's structure, its musculoskeletal and connective tissue systems, reflect and are reflected in, the person's general state of being; primarily physiologically. Many if not most osteopaths would extend this sphere of influence to include mento-emotional and 'spiritual' levels of being too. Whereas any truly holistic conceptual approach would discourage compartmentalisations like this, for now, let's allow these different aspects of the organism to stand as separate areas of study or scrutiny. Indeed, they have to be so at certain stages of study for obvious reasons. (The problem is that, in mainstream medicine, they frequently *remain* separated, and this division is reflected in treatment strategies that are very compartmentalised, but more of this later).

Orthodox physicians and surgeons vary in the extent to which they truly accept this idea. Some claim that it is obvious, in that damaged tissue clearly displays altered form and correspondingly, altered function. Others find the claims for this entire concept strange, the functional melding of 'structure' and physiology remaining an elusive concept that resists any translation into a therapeutic approach.

Meanwhile, let's look at some of the theories underpinning this 'structure/ function' dialogue on which osteopaths (and others in roughly similar fields) base so much of their thinking.

How do structure and function influence one another?

The ideas in question have been through different stages of evolution, in part reflecting the culture of the time and in part reflecting the boldness of the proposer! Strangely, Still's ideas seem even more prescient because theorising went through a rather over-mechanical phase during the first half of the 20th century from which we are slowly beginning to emerge. In his *Textbook of Osteopathy*, Thomas Dummer (1999) describes the evolution to which osteopathy has been subject, breaking it down into the following broad phases:

- 1874–1900/1920: the 'formative' phase
- 1920–1950/60: the 'structural'/mechanical phase
- 1960–1975: the greater emergence of the 'cranial'/'functional' influence
- 1975 onwards: a 'return to source' involving the re-assertion of Holism and Still's principles with an equal emphasis on structural and functional approaches.

The timing of these phases is, of course, approximate but the periods could be said to reflect the culture of the time. The end of the 19th century was ripe for innovation, supporting Still's pioneering and formative ideas. The first half of the 20th century saw a remarkable proliferation and refinement of the products of a mechanical culture that had its roots in the industrial explosion of the 19th century. Consequently, many subtle elusive concepts in osteopathic theory were couched in exaggeratedly mechanical terms using mechanical analogies. This may well have contributed to the enduring tendency to 'over-mechanise' the osteopathic process and along with it, the view of musculoskeletal function.

The second half of the 20th century saw a huge sophistication in the world of electronics and electrical engineering with solid state science and the proliferation of 'machines' whose mechanisms were clean and invisible. A subtlety developed in osteopathic thinking that respected more sophisticated neural and fluid dynamics and less emphasis on the body as a machine whose parts had to be mechanically re-arranged. Paralleling the insinuation of quantum theory into the production of equipment and everyday objects of various kinds and the growth of nanotechnology, some osteopaths began to draw on the fascinating inferences from quantum theory that illuminated aspects of both physiology and technique. These saw a growth of interest in subtler methods of treatment on the part of the public and students/practitioners alike. Coupling this with systems theory, ecology, chaos theory and globalisation, the appeal of holism began to assert itself with greater confidence than ever. It was time to revisit and re-interpret Still's (and Sutherland's) principles and move osteopathy forward *because* of them (not *despite* them, as some would have it).

Generally speaking, different aspects of the 'structure/function' dialogue are given emphasis based on:

a) The particular period in the profession's history
b) The school and school of influence from which you have emerged
c) The approach or orientation with which you feel an affinity, very much based on your own ideas, philosophy, breadth of understanding etc.

Ground Rules and those Structure/Function Bonds

For now, let's run through the basic tenets of the osteopathic method, concepts on which most of the profession would agree (though not quite all!)

In a nutshell, these concepts are based on three fundamental elements: firstly, fluid dynamics; secondly, information transfer and regulation; and thirdly, constitutional vitality. Another way of putting it is that we're dealing with 'fluids, nerves and fields'. All of these, when well-integrated, permit the body to express its potential for self-regulation, health and healing. Furthermore, the effective operation of the tissues that comprise the body structure (along with all other tissue) is intimately interwoven into the function of these three, not necessarily as 'cause' or 'effect' but as 'part'. (It is probably more accurate to think in terms of 'structure' as *being* 'function' when it comes to living tissue, and in that sense, they are virtually inseparable. But we still like to differentiate them to teach the concept, 'structure' being more apparently 'manually accessible'.)

So how does a breakdown in these areas occur? What are the processes that are involved? Well, I suggest the following provides a guide. It summarises the dynamics on which all good osteopathy is based, with parameters that are in a perpetual state of reciprocating function, a state to which the osteopathic practitioner is constantly attuned.

1. 'The rule of the artery is supreme' (Still). The emphasis here is on the importance of a healthy blood supply to the health and vitality of all organs, tissues and structures PLUS the influence that altered structural function can have on this. Incorporated in this principle is the role of the circulatory systems as a conduit for the distribution of nutrients along with the orchestrated and self-regulating biochemical elements that most organisms have the *potential* to produce most of the time.

2. An efficient and unobstructed venous and lymphatic drainage from all tissues and the avoidance of congestive hyperaemic states PLUS the dominant influence of abnormal musculoskeletal and connective tissue states on these.

3. Healthy and integrated musculoskeletal and connective tissue systems incorporating sound tissue texture and tone, well-modulated and distributed mobility throughout the body complete with good functional integration throughout the body structure and framework. More of this later.

4. Sound patterns of body use in terms of locomotion, general mobility and posture and their influence on the above (as well as what follows). For example, the postural elements are significant in producing correct intra-thoracic and intra-abdominal pressures with their effects on circulation and respiration as well as reflecting the means by which we express our relationship with the world through our 'primary machinery of life' (Korr, 1967). This so often mirrors aspects of personality and character.

5. The profound interplay between good structural function and the operation of the central and autonomic nervous systems: musculoskeletal function as reflected in healthy mobility is intertwined with healthy integrated function within the spinal cord and its myriad patterns of reflex operation. These will be expanded on further below. For many, this area has been the crux of their understanding of structural medicine and the notion that disturbed spinal mechanics can be part of a neurally based breakdown in the body that results in abnormal physiology. This was, of course, boldly asserted by the chiropractic profession traditionally: another profession whose tenets became subject to a rather over-simplified interpretation, i.e. that areas of spinal malfunction reflected a spinal malpositioning of a vertebra or vertebrae (the subluxation) that resulted in pressure on nerves causing malfunction in the body's physiology: a graphic, simple and somewhat inaccurate representation of the chiropractic credo. It is interesting that many early osteopaths based their ideas on this simple if implausible model too and many a patient has been fobbed off with this explanation. Still, it's easy to grasp and communicate even if it's largely wrong! We'll look later at the *improved* version of this concept.

6. The structural integrity of the body within which the structural functioning of the entire body is in a state of reciprocity: 'structure affects structure'. This is also profound as different aspects of the structural system, different tissues,

communicate with one another in extraordinary ways. Complex patterns of compensation arise as the body structure responds and adapts to altered stresses and strain patterns. Systems of spinal 'mechanics' have long been a part of the fundamental teaching of osteopathy, from Fryette, Littlejohn, Hall and Wernham, through to the concept of tensegrity (Buckminster Fuller, Donald Ingber, Steven Levin), and its relevance to all connective tissue, and the various theories of 'biotypology' and their perspectives on diagnosis and treatment needs. More of this later too.

7. The *connective tissue* of the body is a unit of function, a matrix subject to the mechanical laws of tensegrity, as stated, and forming the most direct and significant interface between structure and function, down to the level of the cell. This is of central importance; it not only validates Still's emphasis on the 'fascia' as the prime support for healthy physiology – *'By its action we live and by its failure we die'* (Still 1892) – it is also the area within our sphere of study which is most significantly substantiated by remarkable cutting-edge research in biology. This relates to the concept of the body as a matrix of bioelectrical signalling providing a communication network that complements the nervous and circulatory systems. It affords information exchange and transfer from any one part of the body, throughout the entire organism through the quantum mechanical, piezoelectric and semi-conductor properties of living tissue, collagen and water. (Szent-Györgyi, 1957)

8. The 'energetic' matrix that reflects all these things along with its role as a repository for mento-emotional and subtler 'material' in the patient's conscious, unconscious and even 'spiritual' wholeness. (Some find this last a little tricky; allow it to stand for now.) The capacity of the body to store and reflect aspects of the patient's being, their relationship with themselves as well as their world is truly extraordinary, from the commonly observed introverted or arrogant/extraverted postures and patterns of movement, to the storage of emotional (and physical) trauma. Freud himself, steeped in neurology and physiology, said 'the Ego is first and foremost a body Ego'. Though we tend to use this aspect of observation and to refine our perception of it in practice, it is, of course, a part of everyday experience. We respond to all kinds of cues as we interact with others and unthinkingly note their body language, their demeanour, even the 'energy' they transmit to (or drain from) us. We know instantly if we like it, if we're drawn to it or if we find it draining or offensive. 'Energetic' exchange between people is a phenomenon of which we are all aware. The scope to understand it and to explore its potential in a complex form is a beguiling part of the patient–practitioner dialogue or 'dance'.

9. Rhythmicity: a concept with particular significance to osteopaths though often interpreted in different ways. It is manifest in good treatment, in healthy tissue and in the tidal fluctuation of cerebrospinal and extracellular fluids, so vital a part of the 'cranial' concept that encapsulates the vitalistic principle and its

translation into tissue health through the phrase that Sutherland borrowed: 'the breath of life.' Herbert Fröhlich (1988) writes of the property of biological systems to express coherent oscillations. While Alfred Pischinger (2007) speaks of the inherent capacity of rhythmic oscillation in the connective tissue matrix. In various ways, good osteopathic treatment is able to impart or to enhance rhythmicity in living tissue. More of this later too.

To summarise: the osteopathic concept provides a 'map' by which we can navigate a diagnostic and therapeutic route. The principles are related to:

a) An understanding of 'mechanical' interactions in the body framework
b) An appreciation of how 'function' (physiologically, emotionally etc.) is reflected in 'structure'
c) A grasp of the interactive process that is part neural, part circulatory, part 'energetic', involving information exchange in many forms, and the ability to observe, palpate and interpret these primarily in terms of patterns of mobility and motility.

Now, quite evidently, osteopathy is not the first or last discipline to place emphasis on the importance of fluid and information dynamics on health, but what it did and continues to do is to emphasise how often quite subtle disturbances and alterations in them can lead to dysfunction, disease or pathology if they are not dealt with (either through processes of compensation, adaptation or resistance, or through therapeutic aid), and the role of the body structure and its integrated operation in this regard.

Having lived with virtually a century of 'chemical' medicine that has seen research and practice revolutionise patient care in our society, Still's thoughts on drugs will seem misplaced to some. However, he was at pains to emphasise that the body was a master of chemical self-regulation which would follow the process of structural adjustment and reintegration. This principle has held up well in the osteopathic field, but one would obviously caution against the wholesale rejection of the best use of medication and the enormous benefits to patients that this has brought. At the same time, the notion of the efficacy of intrinsic biochemical self-regulation weighs strongly in the balance with the overuse of medication and the iatrogenic sequelae that are all too common. Still's talk of 'God's own drugstore' and the way that its benefits can be activated in perfect integration by osteopathy is as relevant as ever, but many of the achievements of modern pharmacology should be acknowledged too, especially when compared with the comparative unsophistication of the medicine of Still's time. Still's legacy, for osteopaths anyway, has been to adopt a less invasive approach to chemical regulation by stimulating self-regulatory mechanisms through the influence of structural reintegration and its powerful constitutional effects. Such a position really highlights one of the most pertinent contrasts between allopathic and osteopathic cultures.

More on structure/function 'bonds'

So next, we'll need to look at some of these extraordinary 'structure/function' bonds in a little more detail. They provide a model that seems so natural that I often wonder why the osteopathic concept has struggled so hard to gain acceptance. However, some of these areas are supported by remarkable research in fields that are often considered challenging to mainstream orthodoxy. But bear with it.

FLUIDS: BLOOD, LYMPH, WATER

Blood Supply

Still's first principle, 'the rule of the artery is supreme' is clearly a little florid in its way, but its meaning is hardly likely to be unacceptable to anyone. What it clearly states is the self-evident fact that health, healthy tissue and normal function are dependent on a relatively efficient blood supply.

Blood is the carrier of food and oxygen to cells and it is the means by which waste products and the by-products of metabolism are transported to the liver and kidneys. Galen (c. AD 130–c. 200), one of the most distinguished physicians of antiquity, demonstrated that arteries transported blood and not air. But it was not until 1628 and William Harvey that the dynamics of blood flow, with the heart as its pump, enabled a proper understanding of the circulatory system. With its 160,000 km of blood vessels in each human and its 5,000 billion red blood cells being renewed at the rate of 25 million per day by the bone marrow; that's about 300 per second.

But what is important to us here is that such unimpeded arterial operation is potentially affected by 'structural' malfunction. Now this is also self-evident up to a point in that gross structural change or abnormality, deformity and trauma are quite likely to have deleterious effects on circulation. Osteopathy takes this much further though to claim that relatively subtle changes in the motion characteristics in tissue, from osseous intervertebral motion abnormalities to the subtlest oscillatory changes in connective tissue (and even subtler than that) alter fluid dynamics and pressure gradients that can be physiologically highly relevant. These effects can be local e.g. by direct constriction of blood vessels or inflammatory responses, or they may be systemic as in body cavity pressure changes that can produce changes in circulatory pressure. They may relate to local tissue repair and healing, or might have much more generalised significance involving the blood supply to a vital organ. The point here then is not the revelation that blood matters, but the assertion that structural function affects the mechanism of its delivery, its transport, its availability and even its quality.

Drainage: Venous and Lymphatic

There are, of course, countless examples of pathophysiological effects of both local and systemic congestion in the venous and lymphatic systems, from localised swelling and oedema in a limb through to congestion in the renal or cardio-pulmonary networks. Such effects can be serious, even fatal, others might be troubling, many will go unnoticed for years until the effect of such 'stasis' and 'passive hyperaemia' might lead to the gradual downgrading of an organ's vital function, with cyst formation or cellular deterioration; uterine fibroids, for example, being one of thousands of possible consequences. As with the significance of good arterial blood supply, healthy venous and lymphatic drainage provide the complementary part of efficient fluid dynamics on which health depends.

Once again, it is the part that this plays in the totality of body function that includes all of the systems mentioned in this section as an integrated organic whole, along with the network or matrix that encompasses the neurohormonal, musculoskeletal and connective tissue systems. Here, the importance of the mechanical effects, both gross and subtle, of structural balance and patterning or configuration of the body, along with the tension and mobility features of all structural elements, have a profound influence on the fluid dynamics so vital to health.

Water

Most people appreciate that water is essential to life. Indeed many these days won't travel very far without their own portable supply of it. However, the extraordinary properties of this substance that makes up 75-85% of us are largely unrealised by most. For water does not just quench and lubricate. Water 'responds', 'behaves' and 'communicates'. Through the patterning of its hydrogen bonds and many other unique properties, it has a molecular structure that reflects the solutes that it contains and mediates innumerable molecular reactions and transactions in the body. Moreover, its inherent molecular behaviour expresses itself mechanically, electrically and chemically to influence, mediate and govern most, if not all, the body's vital functions. Where many will recognise water's ubiquitous nature, its extraordinary scope of influence is the subject of specialist study, whilst its connection with the rhythmic expression based in the oscillation of tissues and cells is fundamental to osteopathic theory and practice. Paul Lee explores this phenomenon beautifully in his book *Interface: Mechanisms of Spirit in Osteopathy* (2005) which is, in my view, essential reading for students and graduates alike. In it, Lee refers to water's properties of 'life support' through its various remarkable qualities and cites Theodor Schwenk (1996) who enumerates those qualities of metabolism, sensitivity and rhythmicity. And in his Foreword to James Oschman's *Energy Medicine in Therapeutics and Human Performance* (2003), Karl Maret MD eloquently expresses this notion yoking it to Szent-Györgyi's contention that the 'submolecular' or the electronic dimension – generally neglected in biology – be most essentially added to the other prime concerns of the biologist: the macroscopic (anatomy), the microscopic (cells), and the molecular (proteins). Maret writes:

> All living processes in the body depend on the transfer of charges to conduct energy and support life. The entire watery matrix of our bodies is interconnected by complex charge-coupled fields that receive around sixty pulsations of electromagnetic energy from our beating heart each minute. . . . Every cell in the body is in intimate electromagnetic contact with the toroidal-shaped magnetic field of the heart.

Maret comments on the controlling unifying influence that this exerts on the entire connective tissue matrix, the largest *organ* of the body. As we discuss later, the role of the matrix as the mediator of bioelectric and biochemical information is paramount as described in the work of Alfred Pischinger, Robert Becker, and Szent-Györgyi himself. Furthermore, its tensegrous and piezoelectric properties (shared with collagen and water, of course) link it beautifully to the osteopathic 'structure/function' concept, and as stated later in this respect, Donald Ingber's contribution (with the concept of *mechanotransduction*, Ingber, 2008) has been a superb and invaluable contribution to this 'structure/function' bonding so central to our thinking. Furthermore, it is the water that affords the living protein in the body its semi-conductor properties, the assertion of Albert Szent-Györgyi that was erroneously contradicted by his critics' sampling of 'dead' *dehydrated* proteins. This is interesting when coupled with Glen Rein's assertions (*Frontier Perspectives*, 1998*)* that 'certain biomolecules act as superconductors and biological systems in general exhibit non-local, global properties which are consistent with their ability to function at the quantum level' (Del Guidice *et al* 1989, Popp & Chang 1979*)*. As Rein states, little attention has been given to the probability that this behavior can be accounted for by the presence of endogenous quantum fields in biological systems, fields that can influence the body's endogenous electromagnetic fields.

Spinal mobility

We look at the important area of spinal mobility in the next chapter, but no overview of osteopathy would be complete without a mention of what, to many, is central to osteopathic thinking.

Abnormal spinal motion has become the touchstone of palpatory diagnosis in osteopathy (along with other systems of manipulative treatment). Virtually all schools and styles of osteopathic teaching acknowledge the significance of the altered physiology that accompanies restrictions or abnormalities of motion of the vertebrae along with the concomitant changes in muscles and ligaments. The obsolete theory of the vertebral 'osteopathic' lesion as the malpositioned segment(s) placing pressure on nerves and causing physiological effects can only really be redeemed in two types of case: firstly, in the genuinely 'positional' lesion that occurs chiefly as the result of trauma and almost always to the atypical spinal areas (the upper cervical and lumbo-sacral articulations); and secondly, in cases of severe spinal pathology, either traumatic, congenital or degenerative. Most spinal lesions that we are called upon to treat are abnormalities of mobility AND accompanying irritability. This latter is extremely important and it is a vital part of the physiological 'story' of the lesion in all its complexity, both in terms of what sustains it and what it leads to.

Irvin Korr

The understanding of the mechanism of the lesion was advanced hugely by Professor Irvin Korr in the 1940s and 1950s who with Dr J S Denslow and others explored and expanded our knowledge on both of these areas so vital to the osteopathic approach. This is work he was to develop and expand over the next 30 years. For osteopaths, it helped to replace the idea of the lesion as a source of mechanical pressure with the more accurate idea of a focus of raised physiological sensitivity or irritability, an altered physiological state that could potentially produce overstimulation of related neural pathways; a phenomenon known as raised 'facilitation'. Furthermore, Korr was explicit about the ways in which this increased irritability affects all related nerves and their innervated tissues whether they be muscles, blood vessels or viscera via 'autonomic' pathways through somatico-visceral and viscero-somatic reflexes. The creation of this perspective drew wonderfully on Littlejohn's ideas in which the emphasis on the *physiological* effects of structural malfunction was paramount, overriding a purely mechanistic view of spinal function and expanding it into a neurophysiological and biochemical phenomenon. Furthermore, the neural processes that might lead to dysfunction were shown to be multi-directional in terms of both impulse-based and non-impulse-based mechanisms, i.e. processes mediated by the conduction property of nerve impulses and the phenomenon of axonal transport, the distribution of axonal proteins to target tissues whether skeletal or visceral (Korr, 1977).

The mechanisms by which the lesion is generated and sustained were also elaborated by Korr's work on 'proprioception' and the role of the muscle spindles in which the consequences of 'incompatible' data from joint, muscle and tendon receptors bombarding the spinal cord segment were elaborated (Korr, 1967). Along with Richard van Buskirk's writings on the role of 'nociceptors' (1990), a greater understanding of the lesion and the effects and aims of manipulative treatment (of whichever kind) became clarified (Korr, 1977).

As discussed in the chapter on 'reciprocity', the significance of the *unity* of body function can never be over-emphasised, so that the neuromuscular information generated by the lesion states to which I refer creates and sustains a generalised alteration in the patterning of musculoskeletal function as a whole through many mechanisms of compensation, synergy and adaptation. The somatic dysfunctional states exist as multiples that form structural patterns the ingredients of which are prioritised according to a diagnostic system or rationale. But this is only part of the story as the complex web of bioelectrical signalling that pervades all living tissue is based in the function of the connective tissue matrix and its remarkable role in both body function and osteopathic theory. This compounds the structural patterning immensely. However, it is negotiable via both an understanding of the role of the matrix itself and a facility to employ a therapeutic method that engages it, e.g. the 'cranial' osteopathic approach.

The connective tissue matrix

What exactly *is* connective tissue? It is a class of tissue that breaks down into many subtypes or categories but includes virtually every part of what we think of as the body structure or framework including bone, cartilage, membrane, tendon, ligament and the fibres, cells and ground substance that we associate with the extracellular matrix. Rich in collagen and water molecules, it displays the remarkable properties that have come to light with the work of physiologist Albert Szent-Györgyi, physicist Herbert Fröhlich, and MD Alfred Pischinger among others, all of whose work figures repeatedly in these explorations of the osteopathic concept. Many of these features exemplify what Szent-Györgyi considered a major omission in biological science: the bioelectrical 'semi-conductor' properties of living tissue (primarily collagen and water), its piezo-electric properties, and its role as a rapid communication system to complement the nervous and circulatory systems. He proposed that proteins are semi-conductors which can, therefore, be regulated to influence the way they conduct electrons. In fact, this is a property shared by all molecules comprising the extracellular matrix.

This connective tissue matrix in its entirety is, in a sense, 'architectural' as well as 'energetic' and 'informational', and is called 'the living matrix' by Oschman to include the cytoskeletal framework and its relationship to the cell nucleus and its DNA. Furthermore, the information carried by the matrix influences the genetic material in the cell in a 'two-way' fashion suggesting that the cellular DNA does not have primacy in the regulatory function of tissues but is itself modulated by connective tissue matrix function in its communication, transport, energetic and informational roles (Lipton, 2005).

This 'energetic and informational' dimension is remarkable in itself and is supremely important in the way it 'challenges' the perspective of 'gene supremacy' in the approach to living systems. The way that such living systems or life forms become organised to develop their unique characteristics, in other words, the way that life *is,* remains a mystery. However, in 1968, Herbert Fröhlich began to expound on the way that living things express informational 'fields' in the form of electromagnetic waves, and many researchers (famously including Rupert Sheldrake and his work on morphogenic fields) have developed this theme since, whilst Fröhlich's work also looked back to the ideas of researchers like Harold Saxton Burr (Burr, 1957) who began work on 'life fields' in the 1930s. Meanwhile the patterning and functioning of living tissue is quite probably a reflection of the organisation of energetic fields that have been variously conceived by several researchers over many decades, and while all have been subject to rejection or eclipse by establishment 'science', they are still with us; they refuse to go away! Biologist and complexity theorist, Stuart Kauffman, tackles the enigma of 'life' saying that 'organisms are not just tinkered-together contraptions, but expressions of deeper natural laws' (Kauffman, 1995). What's more, the way energy communicates via ionic fluxes created by electrolytes in plasma and tissue fluids switches many biologically active compounds on and off (Roberts, 1997). Interestingly, Still and Sutherland intimated dynamics such as these in their own terms long before biologists elaborated the detail.

RECAP

To recap, the structure of the body as an informational network is far more sophisticated than suggested merely by the neuromuscular reflex and circulatory systems, and, as Still asserted over 100 years ago, involves the fascial and entire connective tissue matrix in fundamental ways:

- Intracellular physiology is dependent on rhythmic 'coherent' oscillatory 'motion', a quality of healthy living tissue (Fröhlich, 1988).
- Cytoskeletal tensegrous formation and function affect the efficiency and quality of information transfer to tubulin polymers and microfilaments comprising the cytoskeleton and their configuration (Hameroff, 1988) and are, in turn, influenced by the signalling mediated by the extracellular matrix. This applies whether we are looking at muscle cells, epithelial cells, immune cells, nerve or bone cells (Ingber, 2008).
- Integrins or integral membrane proteins form a physiological and informational link between the extracellular space and the cell interior, affecting protein metabolism and conformation, even at the cell nucleus and affecting gene expression.
- Molecular information transfer is conveyed through the semi-conductor property of tissues and their crystalline lattice structure or composition (Szent-Györgyi) while it is also subject to motile and tensional qualities exerted on the body through motion and mechanical balance or integrity via the property of piezoelectricity, notably in collagen and water.
- Ultra-fast electronic transfer – in the form of direct current or DC – is a rapid

body-wide function of the perineurium that complements the impulse conduction property of the nervous systems (Becker & Sheldon, 1985).

The extracellular matrix and connective tissue 'system' as a whole comprises a medium through which the body 'structure' directly influences physiology even at the level of the cell – bioelectrically, biochemically and metabolically (Pischinger) and conveys information globally to cells throughout the body at a far greater speed than the neurohormonal and circulatory and reflex networks on their own.

QUANTUM EFFECT

Quantum mechanical principles functionally or conceptually unite energy, mass and information, and have given substance to a view that palpatory 'intention' can direct stimuli to tissues in a pivotal and strategic manner where it can promote 'coherence' (Mae-Wan Ho, 2008) through a process known as 'entrainment' (Oschman, 2003). Furthermore, subtle tactile stimuli specifically and intelligently applied to the body tissues will, through the bioelectrical responsiveness of living tissue, change the body-wide tensegrous arrangement or formation of the connective tissue matrix to impact on structural integrity and its beneficial effects on physiology. This mind/body interplay is highly contentious for many but is worthy of exploration through the work of the researchers whose work Oschman so comprehensively summarises in his texts. We'll look further at this later.

It is worth stating here that, owing to the functional reciprocal operation of the various elements of the body structure, profound connective tissue or fascial changes clearly result from approaches that are predominantly focused on muscle and bone, and vice versa. Minimal highly focused spinal vertebral corrections, for example, have penetrating effects on structural function 'globally' as well as on neurophysiological and circulatory dynamics. Similarly, 'fascial' and 'cranially' oriented approaches effectively alter musculoskeletal reflexes, muscle tone and vertebral mobility. Holistically applied treatment has holistic resonances despite the type of tissues initially targeted.

ADAPTATION

Lest the model I'm presenting is taken too literally to suggest that distortions and abnormalities on any of the foregoing parameters will inevitably lead to malfunction, illness or disease, it is timely here to affirm the universal concept of 'adaptation' as a vital ingredient in the maintenance of health, the overcoming and reversal of these distortions, along with the principle of homeostasis, the tendency of the body to re-assert equilibrium (functionally and mechanically) whenever possible. Indeed, the human body is masterful at adapting to and compensating for many functional abnormalities and disturbances. In fact it was Erwin Schrödinger (1944), the founder of quantum theory, who answered the mystery of 'what is life?' saying that living things are distinguished by the facility to create order from disorder, a sort of reversal of entropy. However, it is where that process fails or is too costly to the physiological (and sometimes psychological) reserves of the individual that an element of 'breakdown' occurs and help is required. These are the patients who come to see us. Perfectly adapted individuals usually don't.

CONCLUSION

So the osteopathic method which was enshrined in Still's dictum that it is 'the law of mind, matter and motion', we might elaborate thus: it is based on the concept of 'structure/function' unity; it is based on the vision of the body as the organisation or orchestration of informational fields reflecting circulatory, neural, biochemical and bioelectric signalling, producing the potential for self-regulation and repair; and finally, that these are accessible through physical (manual) interventions and therapeutic agencies that can be modulated by knowledge and intention.

By and large, the aim of treatment is not so much the confrontation of illness or disease (though many palliative arrows exist in the osteopathic quiver), more the access and stimulation of the vital quality of health and the facilitation of its expression, thereby overcoming many of our patients' problems. The extent to which this can overcome severe health problems is often remarkable, and increasingly osteopaths are now cast in the role of primary healthcare physicians. There is an important question here as to the extent to which osteopaths in the UK can be permitted to fill this role completely owing to their limited access to certain emergency procedures, resources and facilities involving direct access to hospitals and conventional colleagues which some critical situations would require. It is, after all, the access to secondary and tertiary care that allows primary care to be effective in certain circumstances.

Naturally, there will sometimes be limits to the efficacy of our approach, and major pathologies and highly virulent infections can and often do overwhelm the average constitution, even with osteopathic support. However, in a huge proportion of human ills and especially the 80% that tend to be considered 'functional', osteopathic methods can have an astonishing level of effectiveness as patterns of ill health (with their associated multiplicity of symptoms – often attributed erroneously to separate ailments) are reversed or resolved and health once again asserts itself with greater potency.

Caveat

But in case the elegance of this approach should persuade you that it is the ultimate panacea, there are, as in all therapeutic systems, limitations. We are often humbly chastened when confronted with the mysteriously stubborn case; the familiar condition in a patient we consider well-understood and 'read' (or diagnosed), a strong patient/practitioner link with no detectable resistant psychogenic elements, no 'practitioner addiction' and no lurking or overwhelming pathology. And for all the drawing forth of that inner 'healing', the patient continues to struggle. That quest for clear understanding and certainty will, despite all our dedication and insight, remind us that there is always more to know, more perhaps we cannot know, and every model and its exponents have their limits. However, whereas it is essential to know one's limitations and the limitations of one's method, it can be anything but straightforward, for many oft-seen conditions will, as stated, sometimes fail to respond whilst extraordinary and unexpected results sometimes occur with very rare or complex cases. What is more, premature referral can be unwise, both evading the possibility of 'breakthrough' and committing the patient to serial referral, itself destabilising (especially when separation or emotional rejection play a part in the patient's story).

Meanwhile, the principles and the model remain key, for it is only through them that we can hope to access and stimulate our patients' constitutions, to elicit and enhance the inner resource of each individual, their potential and their possibilities in the reclamation of health and wellbeing.

OSTEOPATHIC SCHEMA:

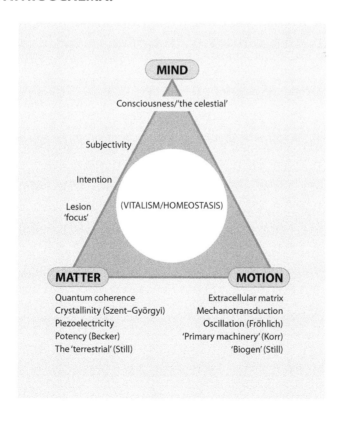

REFERENCES

Becker, R & Sheldon, S, 1985, *The Body Electric: Electromagnetism and the Foundation of Life*, William Morrow & Co.

Burr, H S, 1957, *Yale Journal of Biology and Medicine* 30(3).

Del Guidice, E, 1989, Magnetic flux quantization and Josephson behaviour in living systems, *Physica Scripta* (40), 786.

Dummer, T, 1999, *Textbook of Osteopathy*, Jotom.

Fröhlich, H, 1988, *Biological Coherence and Response to External Stimuli*, Berlin: Springer Verlag.

Fulford, R C, ed Cisler, T, 2003, *Are We On The Path?* The Cranial Academy.

Hameroff, S, 1988, Coherence in the cytoskeleton: Implications for biological information processing. In: *Biological Coherence and Response to External Stimuli*, ed. Fröhlich H, Springer Verlag, 242–263.

Ho, M-W, 2008, *The Rainbow and the Worm*, World Scientific Publishing.

Ingber, D, 2008, Tensegrity and mechanotransduction, *Journal of Bodywork and Movement Therapies* 12:198–200.

Kauffman, S, 1995, *At Home in the Universe*, New York, Oxford University Press.

Korr, I, 1967, *The Physiological Basis of Osteopathic Medicine*. The Postgraduate Institute of Osteopathic Medicine and Surgery.

Korr, I, 1977, *The Neurobiologic Mechanisms in Manipulative Therapy*, Plenum.

Kuhn, T, 1962, *The Structure of Scientific Revolutions*, University of Chicago Press.

Lee, R P, 2005, *Interface: Mechanisms of Spirit in Osteopathy*, Stillness Press.

Lipton, B, 2005, *The Biology of Belief*, Hay House.

Oschman, J, 2003, *Energy Medicine in Therapeutics and Human Performance*, Butterworth-Heinemann.

Pischinger, A, 2007, *The Extracellular Matrix and Ground Regulation*, North Atlantic Books.

Popp, F & Chang, J, 1979, Mechanisms of interaction between electromagnetic fields and living systems, *Science in China* 43:507–518.

Rein, G, 1998, Biological effects of quantum fields and their role in the natural healing process, *Frontier Perspectives* 7:16–23

Roberts, M, 1997, *New Scientist*.

Schrödinger, E, 1944, *What is Life?* Cambridge University Press.

Schwenk, T, 1996, *Sensitive Chaos*, Rudolf Steiner Press.

Still, A T, 1892, *Philosophy and Mechanical Principles of Osteopathy*, republished 1986, Osteopathic Enterprise.

Szent-Györgyi, A, 1957, *Bioenergetics*, Academic Press.

van Buskirk, R, 1990, Nociceptive reflexes and the somatic dysfunction: a model, *Journal of the American Osteopathic Association* 90:792–794, 797–809.

Chapter 2

The vital quality of Motion

When teaching, I was always a fan of the essay in exams and, during the rise of the 'multiple choice' craze, held on to the essay form for the papers I set. I felt that essays would reflect the students' thought processes as they 'joined up the dots', whereas multiple choice simply gave us the dots. So I wrote rather wordy questions at times and used to joke with the students that, if they took the question and merely rearranged the words, they'd probably come up with the answer!

One provocatively phrased example consisted in taking Still's dictum: osteopathy is the law of Mind, Matter and Motion, posing 'Why should we mind so much about the matter of motion?' Clearly, I was interested in students' take on the significance of 'motion' in an osteopathic context, and whilst some of them probably produced model answers, the following is my own effort.

It is probably true to say that even in the often turbulent world of osteopathy, a world wracked with conjecture, debate and frankly, disagreement, the one area we all agree on is the significance of *mobility* in one guise or another. And although it sounds trite, it is mobility in some form, its quality, range and distribution along with various often quite subtle forms of tissue texture and physiological 'expression' that provide the essential diagnostic indicators in practice.

Now this notion on its own is hardly earth-shattering. Scientists from cell biologists to nuclear physicists are alive to the significance of motion. However, in the realm of the bio-sciences, motion is seen as the basis of life. Indeed, it is life's distinguishing feature as the motion of proteins of various types is what generates and perpetuates life with all of its sustaining functions. Furthermore, it is through motion that living things *express* life, whilst it is through specialised forms of visceral 'motion' that our physiology is able to sustain us so that we can *continue* to express life.

I think one might say that the various ways in which the osteopathic concept has been interpreted, leading to all sorts of professional argument, has been partly due to the different qualities of motion considered significant, palpable and accessible, and we'll look at the range or types of mobility that osteopaths consider below.

Meanwhile, the physiologist Professor Irvin Korr, who dedicated decades of research to the exploration of the basis of osteopathy, was remarkably articulate in his many illuminating papers on the subject and spoke of the significance of the body structure – the musculoskeletal system – as the 'primary machinery of life' through which life was 'lived' or expressed (Korr, 1967). In this sense, he went some way towards supporting the primacy of the body structure and its clinical significance to osteopaths (as well as others in similar fields, e.g. chiropractors etc.). As previously illustrated, the musculo-skeletal system is the largest consumer of energy in the body, a point hardly separate from its constant interplay with the entire metabolic arena within the organism.

Now where it starts to get a bit osteopathic is when we begin to look at just why the quality of motion within the body – let's just keep to the musculo-skeletal system for the moment – should have any bearing on anything else. To put it bluntly, why do osteopaths think they can do anything useful at all in the clinical field by restoring good balanced mobility to the body structure? In other words, why are 'structure' and 'function' in the organism so important to one another?

Perhaps it is because I've been closeted in this osteopathic world for so long, but to me it is remarkable that anyone would think otherwise! If the way the body moves – from its cellular oscillations through to its capacity for gross movement – were *not* significant with impact on the entire physiology, I would find it extraordinarily strange.

Staying with the purely 'musculoskeletal' and without getting too subtle for the moment, well-phased, integrated and relatively normal mobility through the spine and the rest of the structure reflects and influences many vital processes from the circulatory, neural reflex and fluctuant fluid dynamics so essential to tissue and cellular health, right down to the subtleties of bioelec-trical signalling from the connective tissues and into the cell via cell membranes and their transmembranous proteins.

In Chapter 1, we looked at some of the concepts espoused by osteopaths in relation to this complex structure/function dialogue and why, with often more incomplete knowledge than now, osteopaths have successfully treated 'function' (physiology) through 'structure' as well as 'structure' through 'struc-ture', this latter being much closer to the stereotypical view of osteopathy and marginally easier for even the sceptic to concede (the realm of back, neck and extremity pain, etc.).

But now let us look at the various aspects of motion that we assess and interpret in practice and, as we'll see, it is the *integration* of mobility that reflects and sustains the mechanisms of health rather than localised and discreet movements in particular areas. Or to put it more holistically, each localised area of dysfunctional mobility is both a reflection of, and is reflected in, the motion patterns of the body as a whole. Relative motion is the key to understanding the significance of mobility to the health of the organism and without this perspective, we are reduced to a rather linear view along with a somewhat limited influence therapeutically.

Abnormal structural function, then, is expressed through altered patterns of movement, from the gross to the subtle. Traditionally, such phenomena have been termed 'osteopathic lesions' and because the word 'lesion' has particular connotations in conventional medicine, the term has largely been replaced by the more cumbersome 'somatic dysfunction'. (Some of us still prefer the old version.)

THE LESION

In conventional medicine, the term 'lesion' is used to define pathological tissue change in various guises. But in osteopathy, the term 'lesion' or 'osteopathic lesion' has a more functional connotation. Thus it defines altered function, in terms of motion or mobility, texture, resilience, responsiveness or irritability in any tissue but most especially in 'structural' tissues – connective tissue in its broadest sense. Historically this feature has been focussed particularly on the spine, spinal column and associated tissues and has placed emphasis on the quality and range of intervertebral motion. Abnormalities in this respect constitute both localised and generalised physiological changes that sit within cycles of altered physiology involving reflex and informational exchanges between the cranio-spinal structures (and their mechanisms) and associated visceral, neural and circulatory elements. These interactions are subject to the principles elucidated in the section on 'structure/function bonds' in the previous chapter, and not only express alterations in structural mechanics but more importantly reflect and involve complex physiological (neural and biochemical) changes too in which the entire functional arena of the area is altered. Such lesions do, of course, interact in reciprocating fashion to provide patterns of dysfunction that we fashion into a diagnosis, but such patterns are reflective of the interplay of all the functional dimensions that we discussed earlier and that constitute the patient 'persona' in clinical and more general constitutional terms.

Osteopathically, then, we are saying that there is a spectrum of motion expressed in living organisms in their structural and visceral anatomy. Some of it is gross or conspicuous: locomotion, exercise, joint and musculoskeletal movements generally, respiratory motion; some is less conspicuous, at least some of the time, e.g. peristaltic motion, circulatory dynamics, fluctuant motion, so-called 'tidal' motion as conceived within the 'cranial' osteopathic concept, cellular oscillation, molecular movement and right down to the inferred motion of sub-atomic particles and the expression of force fields with their own frequencies and wave-like properties.

These various forms of movement are generally considered important for the expression of organic life (from the gross to the cellular to the molecular) and the sustaining of life processes, such that the idea – not exclusive to osteopathy but certainly central to it – that normal levels of mobility are essential to good physiology is a comfortable one for most people. The notion that really unifies 'structure' and 'function' and truly reflects the saying that 'structure' is *solidified* 'function' (Frymann, 1998) has to be underpinned by an emphasis on integration; motion needs, within certain limits anyway, to be integrated, co-ordinated, phased and patterned, and this criterion is fundamental to the osteopathic view to a considerable degree.

The subtlety and complexity of this 'relative' motion and the extent of its influence physiologically is exemplified in the 'cranial' approach but is by no means exclusive to it. However, it is in the realm of motion as expressed within the 'cranial' concept that osteopathic in-fighting has enjoyed some of its most sporting moments!

Let it be said, at this point, that abnormalities of motion, as with compromises of all sorts within the body, are qualities to which the organism can adapt, so that reasonable levels of health can often be sustained in the presence of altered or disturbed mobility. But this is true throughout all discussions of health: it is the exaggerated levels of 'breakdown' or the excessive deviations from the norm and the necessary compensation required in certain cases – the ultimate failure to cope – that leads to the expression of dysfunction and illness.

We have moved on from a look at the fact that detailed, complex, integrated motion is important to health to a look at the quality of motion itself.

At the highly conspicuous end of the spectrum then, we have locomotion and patterns of body use, so ingeniously encapsulated in the work of F. M. Alexander. Here, the extraordinary way that the concept of 'direction' is taught and instilled in the pupil is as unique as it is inspired, and the benefits to poise, movement and indeed health are there to see in countless teachers and pupils of the Alexander Technique (Alexander, 1910).

When we look at joint and healthy musculoskeletal function generally, we are all mostly aware of the benefits to health and wellbeing that these bring both in terms of physical comfort, psychological habitus, stress reduction as well as such benefits as improved cardiovascular function and other physiological spin-offs; precisely the goals of those keen on sport and exercise.

Patterns of respiration are interesting not least for the obvious benefits to healthy and comfortable breathing and adequate oxygenation, but also for their influence on a healthy O_2/CO_2 balance, metabolism and energy production, as well as the 'massaging' effect on the circulation and viscera of good respiratory excursion and healthy intrathoracic/intra-abdominal pressures. In this sense, altered patterns of breathing can have profound effects on both 'structure' and physiology way beyond that of the respiratory system itself, with direct and indirect influences on, for example, intracranial circulation, the cardiovascular system, gastro-intestinal functioning , peripheral circulation and much else besides.

Let's look next at the link between musculoskeletal mobility (and integrated spinal motion) and the health at the spinal segment with its neural and circulatory corollaries. This is probably the area most familiar to osteopaths and their patients and is the most quoted 'structure/function bond' in traditional osteopathic thinking. We have looked at this in the previous chapter but it is worth reiterating that integrated intersegmental mobility throughout the spine is highly conducive to healthy integrated neural and circulatory function, both locally and systemically. As Professor Korr put it so eloquently, the dysfunctional spinal segment as evidenced by aberrant mobility is like 'the soldier out of step' in an otherwise perfectly drilled brigade; he is not only conspicuous, but he causes trouble; he disturbs everyone around him and therefore threatens to destroy the patterning of the whole group (Korr, 1976). Turning away from the parade ground and back to the spine, this potentially disturbs the spinal mechanics as a whole as well as local physiology, creating a region of increased irritability or 'raised facilitation'. Here, the segment – (this includes all related tissues and their nerve and circulatory elements) – becomes prone to neural overactivity (irritability), as stimuli from any source in the body can potentially 'activate' the segment further as its functional threshold is lowered (Korr, 1967). This whole process constitutes a physiological 'event' in that many biomechanical, biochemical and bioelectrical changes accompany this phenomenon to make the osteopathic lesion a sort of 'micropathology' rather than the simple 'bone out of place' so often imagined. Altered reflex activity involving *proprioceptive* and *nociceptive* sensory pathways serves to sustain this situation of altered function to become one ingredient in the 'total lesion' to which we so often refer. The phenomena of altered proprioception and nociception are instrumental in generating and sustaining the lesion producing connective tissue, circulatory, visceral and immunological changes and the raised facilitation that we associate with the 'somatic dysfunction' or 'osteopathic lesion', as the neural information centring on the relevant spinal segment(s) becomes discordant. Above all, it is important to understand that malfunction of body structures, often without pathology but manifesting a disturbance of motion (either gross or subtle), is a complex physiological process or 'event', often with far-reaching consequences clinically.

The restoration of good segmental mobility – sometimes in a simple and 'local' form – can be enough to make considerable differences to physiological functioning, re-establishing equilibrium in somatico-visceral, viscera-somatic and somatico-somatic neural pathways. However, in most cases, this is insufficient without adequate consideration of the *context* in which this localised spinal lesion expresses itself, in other words, the broader structural and physiological patterning of the patient as a whole. In practice, the significance of this context cannot be over-emphasised. Meanwhile, considerable emphasis is also placed, in osteopathic training, on spinal mobility and 'laws' of motion that were articulated for all time by H. H. Fryette in *The Principles of Osteopathic Technique* and which gave rise to a diagnostic categorisation as well as a prescription for corrective technique and the 'reversal' of the spinal structural lesion or dysfunction (Fryette, 1954). These laws would explain intervertebral function and malfunction, giving a theoretical basis to the aetiology of abnormal spinal configurations and a methodological basis for manipulative correction.

Meanwhile, the holistic model and the significance of 'whole body' patterns along with the context that these provide, should not detract from the changes in physiological dynamics that are often triggered by abnormal segmental function in the spine as well as discreet areas of dysfunction in other body tissues. These may call for more localised palliative measures that can be of lasting benefit. With or without this contextual pattern, the direct pathway(s) of symptom expression have still to be acknowledged and addressed. At this point, the suitability of a 'linear' rather than holistic approach (or vice versa) can be decided. As a rule though, the linear process (of simple cause and effect) is properly seen enfolded in a contextual pattern to enable a treatment strategy that incorporates both palliative and the constitutional objectives.

Finally, it is, of course, essential to remember that inter-segmental spinal motion (and its disturbances) are functionally inseparable from neuromuscular function generally which, along with the entire connective tissue system, form an interface with all aspects of body physiology. Herein, one can find reflections of many aspects of the patient's condition, constitution and potential, this being the osteopath's job based on the application of theory and principle.

THE 'CRANIAL' DIMENSION

And so to the joys of controversy and one of the most extraordinary developments in osteopathy and, in my view, in the practice of medicine: the application of the 'cranial' osteopathic concept.

In this chapter, we are concentrating on motion, so what of 'cranial' motion? If you give yourselves a sneak preview to page 79 in Chapter 5, you can quickly look at Sutherland's 'five phenomena' and see that the common theme amongst these is on the subject of motion. And it is this 'cranial' motion, this subtle form of oscillation (or what Sutherland called 'the breath' or 'the breath of life' to borrow his biblical analogy), that extends throughout the body to all tissues, structures and cells carrying with it the vitality that sustains them. It is this quality of motion that has often lost osteopaths friends, even amongst their own (just as the concept of *vitalism* has sometimes lost osteopaths friends everywhere else!) For, though we use the model of structural motion to teach and learn cranial osteopathic skills, for me, the debate will always hinge on whether, to the analytical mind, what we *feel* as movement is in fact the best effort of our sensory and cognitive apparatus to respond to the awareness and interpretation of a 'field' or 'fields' of function and the complex details of their expression throughout the body tissues via patterns of bioelectrical or electromagnetic signalling.

Cranial work has been practised to good effect for several decades by many who are as unaware of the role that quantum theory might play as they are uninterested. Indeed, as Nicholas Handoll points out so well in his *Anatomy of Potency* (2000), we may never fully comprehend precisely the anatomy of the 'motion' we seem to feel, any more than we can get used to the idea that the sense of 'touch' and experience of solidity are simply the coming together of two or more electromagnetic force fields. However, the detail, the location anatomically, the quality, the health or otherwise of what we *can* feel is as much about motion, its amplitude, direction and nuance as it needs to be for us to 'read' the patient through these 'motion' patterns and have access to the patient's health through them. What's more, the therapeutic interventions unquestionably change the quality of tissue states discernible by both patient and practitioner, and these impact hugely on patients' experience of their own body awareness as well as their states of wellbeing and health.

What remains, however, is firstly *what* is the nature of this perceived motion and secondly, *where* does it come from? All attempts to explain it seem to have been based on speculations about its source. The origin of this movement, whether we call it primary respiration, the fluctuation of the fluid tide, the rhythmic expression of the 'breath of life', or the cranial rhythmic impulse, has exercised the minds of osteopaths since the work came into being, and an interesting division arises between those who would seek its origin within the body – rather like the cardiovascular pulse or the rhythm of respiration – and those who would see it as a reaction to, or transduction of, something extrinsic. This subject was explored as part of a comparative study of views in an article by Andrew Ferguson *et al* in *The Journal of Bodywork & Movement Therapies* (1998). In the article, I placed my own contribution in the latter camp and in so doing subscribe to the idea that organisms express vitality as a product of their interaction with their biosphere, their environment. This, I am aware, is an unfashionable view, since physiological processes are more comfortably explained in terms of intrinsic mechanisms such as Upledger's 'pressurestat' theory (Upledger & Vredevoogd, 1983) or the rhythmic oscillations based on the 'Traub-Hering-Meyer wave' relating to cyclical variations in arterial and venous pressures. But these theories exclude the feasibility of composite fluctuating processes working in unison, as well as the interplay and influence of extrinsic biologically relevant forces acting on the organism to produce these intrinsic observable rhythms.

In the same way, I would assert that the perceived expression of the rhythm is also a product of the interplay or interaction of the patient and practitioner and their respective 'fields'. And this is why we cannot expect the cranial rhythm of any given patient to express itself identically when examined by different practitioners. The practitioner's biological and intentional 'fields' link with the patient in a unique and potent way. The potential for this interaction to render significant therapeutic change has been explored experimentally by Glen Rein (Rein, 1998), William Tiller (Tiller, 1997), and others in their explorations of scalar and quantum fields and the 'particulate and wave space'. Meanwhile its pivotal influence when anchored to the therapeutic model as in osteopathy is demonstrated every day in thousands of treatment sessions that incorporate the method.

But next a look at a few of the theories that have attempted to explain the *intrinsic* origin of this motion. In my opinion, the phenomena described are *manifestations* or expressions of this motion rather than descriptions of what generates it. And here we again get close to one of those subjects that many in science love to hate: *vitalism* – the notion that there exists an inexplicable force that generates a quality we call 'life' which then expresses itself through the many established processes and mechanisms that we *can* analyse.

Osteopaths are not alone in this view. In many areas of science, the attempt to shun vitalism once and for all is proving difficult, as the 'spark' that ignites, energises or expresses the life force continues to be elusive (Brooks, 2010). Meanwhile, it is, I feel, important to emphasise that the 'cranial rhythm', the 'cranial rhythmic impulse' or 'primary respiration' (whichever you prefer) is not the *generator* of life or vitality; it is the reflection or expression of it, and what's even more significant to us in practice, it is accessible.

Force

In the end, it is likely that the basis of the force that energises living organisms will continue to elude us for some considerable time yet. However, I feel it interesting to consider the ubiquity of this energetic force or 'potency' expressing itself through all living things where it becomes transmuted in ways that become 'species-specific' as well as 'tissue-specific'. When motion and vitality express themselves in different living structures, they 'wear' different qualities depending on whether we are considering different parts of the 'structural' system: bone, ligament, muscle, fascia, fibre, fluid, cell, or whether we are looking at nerve tissue or the parenchymal cells of the viscera. Setting aside the functional movements or dynamics of these various structures, the resonances within the tissues themselves have a quality that reflects the type of tissue being considered and its embryological origins.

It is this area of tissue resonance that reflects the state of vitality of the tissues themselves aside from their level of functioning or operation. The latter is what is commonly used in conventional medical assessment. The former is where osteopaths like to focus much of their attention.

The differential point is that the tissue quality is not a product of the tissues themselves but a manifestation of how well the tissues transmute what we call vitality. (An analogy might be the way the body assimilates the vitality in food and, in its metabolism and the use of such fuel, transmutes that vitality into physiological functionality).

It is precisely because tissues express the transmuted 'energy' specifically, reflecting morphological and genetic differences in make-up, that we tend to ascribe the types of motion to the inherent potential of the tissues themselves ignoring the fact that the 'engine' still needs fuel; without it, it is inert.

However, when considering osteopathic correction of these variously expressed motion patterns, their qualitative differences can be important depending on whether the *dominant* restrictions are intervertebral (apophyseal or facet joints), in rib articulations, in ligaments, muscles or membranes, in sutures (i.e. interosseous), within bone (intraosseous), before AND after ossification, or in fluid dynamics or 'fluctuation'. And we haven't even touched on appendicular or visceral motion.

Becker's storm

Although many may not have realised it at the time, in 1963, Rollin Becker DO published the first of five articles in the American Academy of Osteopathy Yearbook that was truly ground breaking when he came up with an extraordinary notion. In describing the patterning of the patient's 'total lesion' in a way that transcended the physician's ability to 'know' definitively what the patient presented clinically, he removed the sense of certainty from the physician's tool box and entreated us to 'listen' to the patient's tissues in a new way where we might eavesdrop on what the patient's body 'knows the problem to be'. In this way, we were invited to marry our own clinical knowledge, with its limitations, to the body's definitive state of 'knowing'. This humble position would pay huge dividends in the creation of a more complete and relevant diagnosis through a refinement of palpation that is key to good osteopathy.

But more importantly perhaps, he introduced the notion that the 'pattern' of the total lesion was largely 'energetic' in nature – rather like a storm or hurricane, and that the 'storm' has an 'eye', centre or focus that harnesses the storm's power, potency or electromagnetic energy. Palpation could permit the physician to read the body's disturbance or disease in terms of such patterning, along with its centre of power which was made available to the practitioner via the use of an intelligent 'fulcrum' (Becker 1997; see Chapter 7). How interesting was this echo of the principles that we were to borrow from the 'quantum' realm and the likes of Albert Szent-Györgyi and Herbert Fröhlich. More than one practitioner who approached Rollin Becker with questions about the 'cranial' mechanism and its basis would be told, 'read quantum physics!'

Bradbury – Dummer – SAT

Meanwhile, in the 1950s, Parnell Bradbury who had trained in both osteopathy and chiropractic, had developed an idea (partly as an expedient) that was expanded remarkably by Thomas Dummer during the 1960s to become his formulation of 'Specific Adjusting Technique' (SAT), one of the basic principles of which was that the structural lesion pattern had, at any one moment, a mechanical focus – a 'primary' – that held the pattern together as its energetic focal point. The release of this focus, when appropriate and performed in a particular way (that involved the practitioner's *conception* of the lesion AND its contextual significance), would permit the pattern to begin a process of resolution. Inherent in both models (Becker's and Dummer's) is the propensity of the body to re-gain the potential to self-regulate by removing patterns that inhibit or obstruct it; one of the many expressions of homoeostasis.

The parallels between these two models, though remarkable, have rarely been celebrated, but they are, for some, fundamental to their approach. But whether conceived as 'energetic' or mechanical or a fusion of the two, the idea of a focal point in the picture is invaluable to a system that can be minimally interventionist and precise whilst calling on the patient's body's own healing responses and their quality of perfect orchestration. Such an integrated reaction is rarely something that can be imposed from without; it is elicited from within provided the therapeutic input is precisely chosen and 'appropriately' addressed, this largely being the result of intellectual analysis, sensitive 'listening' palpation and intention. Both 'cranial' technique and SAT manipulation share these qualities though they do, of course, differ in other ways.

In summary, the key point in this chapter is the significance of motion in the body, particularly of the structural tissues, but in fact more accurately of the entire body in the form of an orchestrated resonance, oscillation or the summation and patterning of various oscillations or rhythms. It is also important that we move beyond the notion of gross movement to include movement qualities that are the subtle 'energetic' expressions of vital function or physiology if you prefer, and the bioelectric dimension. But as with the more conspicuous or gross mobility patterns that we seek to integrate through treatment, the subtler motility patterns can also be 'harmonised' to restore *coherence* ('quantum coherence') in tissues and throughout the entire connective tissue 'matrix' of the body as a whole. This phenomenon, so eloquently expressed and articulated by Mae-Wan Ho (Ho, 2008) is a fundamental piece of the osteopathic jigsaw and builds on Herbert Fröhlich's theories on biological oscillations to produce a vital plank of modern osteopathic theory. We look at both of these later but for now, I'd like to conclude with Oschman's reference to physicist Guido Preparata's provocatively forward-looking extract from *QED Coherence In Matter* (1995) which alludes to a dimension that many consider has been absent from the biological sciences for too long, but which curiously and holistically draws 'mind, matter and motion' into the coherent notion that Still proclaimed:

> *'Quantum electrodynamics is a cornerstone of modern chemistry and condensed-matter physics and thus is the ultimate foundation for current theories of almost all phenomena perceived by the senses, as well as many biological processes and perhaps even consciousness itself.'*

REFERENCES

Alexander, F M, 1910, *Man's Supreme Inheritance*, Centreline Press.

Becker, R, 1963, Diagnostic touch: its principles and application, *Academy of Applied Osteopathy Year Book*.

Becker, R, 1997, *Life in Motion*, Rudra Press.

Bradbury, P, 1967, *The Mechanics of Healing*, Peter Owen.

Brooks, M, 2010, *Thirteen Things That Don't Make Sense*, Profile Books.

Dummer, T, 1995, *Specific Adjusting Technique*, Jotom.

Ferguson, A, Upledger, J, McPartland, J, Collins, M, Lever, R, 1998, Cranial osteopathy and cranio-sacral therapy: current opinions, *Journal of Bodywork & Movement Therapies* 2:28–37.

Fryette, H H, 1954, *The Principles of Osteopathic Technique*, Academy of Applied Osteopathy.

Frymann, V M , 1998, *The Collected Papers of Viola M. Frymann*, American Academy of Osteopathy.

Handoll, N, 2000, *Anatomy of Potency*, Osteophathic Supplies Ltd.

Ho, M-W, 2008, *The Rainbow and the Worm*, World Scientific Publishing.

Korr, I, 1967, *The Physiological Basis of Osteopathic Medicine*, The Postgraduate Institute of Osteopathic Medicine and Surgery.

Korr, I, 1976, The spinal cord as organizer of disease process, *Journal of the American Osteopathic Association* 76:35–45.

Nelson, K E, Sergueef, N, Lipinski, C L, Chapman, A, Glonek, T, 2001, The cranial rhythmic impulse related to the Traube-Hering-Mayer oscillation: comparing laser-Doppler flowmetry and palpation. *Journal of the American Osteopathic Association* 101:163–173.

Preparata, G, 1995, *QED Coherence in Matter*, World Scientific Publishing Co.

Rein, G, 1998, Biological effects of quantum fields and their role in the natural healing process, *Frontier Perspectives* 7:16–23.

Tiller, W, 1997, *Science and Human Transformation*, Pavior Publishing.

Upledger, J & Vredevoogd, J, 1983, *Craniosacral Therapy*, Eastland Press.

Chapter 3

Holism and the osteopathic 'lens'

These days, many people like the idea of 'holism'. It seems to incorporate the notion of completeness, thoroughness and comprehensiveness. But in truth, it's a difficult concept to really get to know. Our culture is one based largely on 'materialism' or a materialistic pragmatism that is itself based on the process of *upward causation* (Goswami, 1993). In other words, notions of reality are constructed out of a summation of what is known and can be pieced together: a reductionist concept that purports to understand things based on an analysis of their component parts. Goswami eloquently contrasts this with its opposite, a form of *idealism* based on *downward causation* and the primacy of consciousness, an overarching enigmatic quality that presides over an unknowable totality, a totality within which the 'gaps', the mysteries and unknowable uncertainties are filled by principles and models, belief systems and faith. Holism dwells within this latter paradigm, a paradigm in which the nature or quality of the 'whole' (always greater than the sum of the parts), is accessed through principles and negotiated by models, and while enticing, it remains enigmatic.

The first premise of holism is that the elements of 'the whole' interact and in so doing, produce something very different from – and greater than – the mere sum of its ingredients, displaying qualities that are unlike those of the parts themselves. This applies to innumerable living and non-living things and all natural phenomena. The human body is, of course, a prime example.

Those of a holistic persuasion look at what connects things and see it as important as the things themselves. And so, it would appear that the spaces between things are not empty but are full of information, and the information contains elements that represent and sustain just what it is that relates the things to one another.

Definition

Perhaps it is because of the insecurity at the heart of human nature that we crave *definition;* it's part of the way we control and relate to things. And as language provides the ultimate means to classify, we are prone to an over-dependence on definition for our conception of reality. In so doing, we mistake description for experience. The act of defining creates a process of 'minimising' and circumscribing which unavoidably de-contextualises and therefore distorts. (The process of de-contextualising removes things from their milieu or their context and those relationships that give things meaning.) So the entire process of analysis and definition provides us with the illusion of greater knowledge (and control too) whilst robbing us of a truer understanding. Clearly, if we only look at our world through a 'microscope', we not only miss out on the larger perspective, we also glean a limited view of what we have examined so meticulously. Such a scenario brings to mind Werner Heisenberg's assertion that things only have meaning *in relationship*; in other words, only in the respect to which they interact with other things. 'The world thus appears as a complicated tissue of events in which the connections of different kinds alternate or overlap or combine and thereby determine the texture of the whole.' (Heisenberg, 1958.)

The culture of materialism and linearity

The scientific revolution of the 16th century not only shifted thinking further away from the subjective, it instilled an obsession with the idea of *certainty* as a distinct possibility, a by-product of intellectual enquiry along with an almost 'linear' pragmatism. This carried with it the implication that, not only did phenomena manifest the process of *cause and effect*, but that there were also *prime* causes; causes that had an almost sovereign role in the creation of certain effects. Though not universal, this attitude has prevailed in medicine (and in our culture) to a considerable degree. Germ theory and the conviction that prime causes of infectious disease reside with micro-organisms, along with enormous advances in genetics research, have both encouraged this position whilst undoubtedly contributing impressively to medical theory and practice. Once an ingredient in a pathophysiological process has been identified and named, there is a tendency to afford it causal primacy whether it be a micro-organism, a gene or the result of virtually any kind of clinical test, from X-ray to scan to blood analysis. Definitive findings take precedence over 'process', even if in reality they account for a small percentage of the overall cause of a problem. I would also argue that this type of thinking has penetrated so-called 'alternative' fields too even where practitioners have *purported* to be 'holistic'. It is as if this preoccupation with singular causes has become the primary object of the diagnostic quest. Even within osteopathy itself, we speak, often misleadingly, of 'primary and secondary lesions', a concept that is useful but which needs careful qualification. This whole issue of causal primacy needs careful consideration. Meanwhile, it should be remembered that eventually even Pasteur asserted *'le terrain est tout'*, a position held over the years by most in the alternative medical field where so-called 'causes' came to be seen as elements *within a context* that permitted their proliferation or expression. This idea has been echoed many times of course; medical anthropologist, Cecil Helman (2006) paralleled the western notion that the body is invaded by bacteria and viruses with the indigenous idea of spirit possession and, in clinical terms, the consequent removal of responsibility from the self.

THERAPEUTICS

The basis of a disciplined approach that includes a holistic therapeutic method is twofold: the first is a principle that most in the field share and that is the conception of the body as a matrix of interlocking and interwoven elements and functions. The second is more elusive but, to my mind, essential: it is the importance of the methodical identification of points of 'access' (therapeutic-ally) that have maximum functional significance to the entire pattern created by those elements and functions. In other words, how do we find and treat the 'whole' through the 'part(s)'? Well, the method has to be based on a model that comprises certain conceptual ingredients. In osteopathy, these ingredients create the facility to interpret data through 'structure' and to access its effects as if looking and working through a 'lens' which focusses to provide a diagnostic interpretation. At its best, such a method contains elegance, economy, beauty and precision. In most circumstances, these qualities allow the practitioner to 'call upon' the patient's own potential to heal in a highly complex and orchestrated manner. We look more at this later, but in practice, this facility arises not so much as a result of a prescribed method, but more as the product of the assimilation of multiple factors, and it is this assimilation that is really the basis of the material in this book.

The 'problem' with Holistic Paradigms (inside as well as outside Osteopathy)

But holism is not without problems when we try to incorporate it into a culture heavily based on the 'materialist' paradigm. Our culture increasingly attempts to define 'quality' in terms of 'quantity'; it examines subtlety and expresses it 'numerically'. The era of information technology encourages this method of evaluation: quantification, 'box-ticking'; a binary, digital world indeed in which 'certainty' is vastly preferred to 'possibility'.

Unfortunately, our profession is in danger of 'modernising' by following this trend (one now definitely favoured throughout the professional and commercial worlds), and would reduce many aspects of patient care – ideally tailored to the individual – to the status of standardised measurable procedures with their outcomes (or targets) similarly evaluated or even demanded. Whilst this might meet a need for greater regulation and control (and security) in our world, it is no way to practise health care.

Meanwhile, holistic paradigms can be a problem, and for two main reasons:

1. Their methods are hard to 'measure', and attempts are usually made to validate them using techniques that belong to other (non-holistic) traditions.
2. They can be 'counter-cultural' whilst still attempting to expand the boundaries

of existing knowledge. Hence they will not conform perfectly or completely to the body of established knowledge or fact. They don't 'fit in.'

Innovative and 'alternative' methods of health care are by definition inevitably and conspicuously at odds with mainstream methods. If they are to be evaluated constructively, a process of evaluation has to be evolved that can resonate with the underlying principles and conceptual form or flavour of the discipline concerned. For this reason they are extremely difficult to measure using more conventional reductionist and 'evidence-based' methods. The inevitable failure of such attempts has led to much negative and unhelpful comment.

In this regard, it has been regrettable that complementary and alternative medical disciplines have attracted so much derision from 'experts' with little or no training in or understanding of the field they've chosen to denigrate. And when, for example, 'placebo' is glibly proffered as the explanation for patient benefit, it should be remembered that such effects are as likely to occur in conventional medicine too with its established culture of authority and its technical prowess. (See Chapter 10.)

It is, then, extremely difficult to evaluate a holistic discipline from a non-holistic perspective even when broad objectives are inevitably shared between conventional and 'alternative' medical models. Sadly though, in this area, prejudices do abound, based, as ever, on poor logic. Countering these negative opinions, the 'alternative' lobby continues to assert the need for *its* methods, with critical comment of its own: for example, that in 2001, the US government published the shocking statistic that conventional medical treatment in the USA is responsible for over 780,000 deaths per year, whilst the *New Scientist* claimed that 80% of medical procedures have never been adequately tested (Abramson, 2005). Now, it should be conceded that the mainstream of medicine is in the front line of treatment in the majority of critical cases, but even so, despite all criticisms, the record for most alternative holistic systems comes nowhere near reflecting such worrying figures.

INTEGRATION

The biosciences contain enough information to underpin the fundamental tenets of osteopathic medicine and to support much of the theory of effectiveness of its therapeutic methods. The principles on which it is based, as outlined in Chapter 1, for example, that the function of the body's structural elements fundamentally affects its physiological function, down to the level of the cytoskeleton and cell nucleus, are demonstrable and verifiable (Pischinger, 2007; Pienta & Coffey, 1991; Ingber, 1998). But the fact that they are not resonant with the conventional medical approach, while in no way diminishing their importance, might well reflect the 'problem with holism' in this context and the prospect of integrating the two contrasting perspectives on healthcare.

For all its extraordinary achievements, the integration of allopathic medicine with holistic methods is difficult though desirable in principle. If we think about it for a moment, it is hard to subsume a holistic approach under an allopathic 'umbrella', whereas the opposite is conceptually feasible. However, the structure of medical practice and the dominance of the allopathic model in the UK and many other 'western' nations make this organisationally impossible.

Objective Trials

The double-blind randomised clinical trial and so-called 'evidence-based' methods of evaluation, so central to medical orthodoxy, are both somewhat inadequate when assessing osteopathic (and other holistic systems of) medicine, and this is for two main reasons:

- Every patient–practitioner exchange is focussed on the unique 'patterning' that gives rise to any particular symptom, syndrome or clinical presentation and in which certain features *only* are held in common, but in which the physiological, psychological, pathological and genetic 'context' are uniquely expressed.
- Clinical intervention is based partly on objectifiable data, but more particularly on the clinician's interpretation of, and interaction with, the complex web or meshwork of interdependent ingredients that create the patient's individual health pattern and disease expression. Furthermore, this interpretation is, in part, subjective, based on the clinician's knowledge (which can never be absolute), experience, technical orientation and skill.

The application of treatment is, then, a craft and a skill. As with surgery, these factors vary between practitioners. They are not – along with surgical procedures – 'standard products', except in fundamental or rudimentary respects. (Think of the features that distinguish a great surgeon from a competent one.)

Meanwhile, a fundamental difference in conceptual orientation resides in the fact that conventional allopathic medicine is primarily based on the attempts to reverse identified malfunctions and confront any agent that threatens health; whereas holistic methods attempt to promote systemic and tissue 'coherence' and functional integration so that the body can intrinsically regain its self-regulatory potential in order to effect both these states, i.e. the reversal of malfunction *and* a heightened resistance to those threatening agents, whether they be pathogens (bacteria, etc.) or any other stressors. These are diametrically opposed conceptual positions. Osteopaths, for example, do not primarily select a technique for each pathophysiological situation (except in certain palliative cases), while this *will* often be the allopathic position, with all its strengths and pitfalls. Osteopaths, on the other hand, essentially address the 'specific' via the systemic and so their priorities, their 'specifics', are completely different, being particular to the individual patient, not merely to the condition itself.

So to summarise, the uniqueness of each patient–practitioner exchange makes evaluation of *method* difficult to research. However, we have a responsibility to establish more appropriate systems of evaluation. We also need to resist the temptation to proscribe methods and scope of practice based on the 'wrong' methods of evaluation. This would be to stultify the practice of osteopathy and to discount its traditional wisdom. Progress should be about ways of revealing this wisdom in greater depth and detail rather than claiming, as some have, that this would drive osteopathy backwards; for this would be to miss the point completely whilst indulging a need to adopt a contemporary methodology for its own sake. Many areas in our society are similarly afflicted where 'best practice' seems to lag streets behind new and developing insights. Perhaps, in a small way, osteopathy might contribute to a tide of change. Unfortunately though, the culture of organisation, regulation and control are in danger of defining our very practices and disciplines, diminishing them in the service of a bureaucratic imperative.

HOLISM VS MULTIFACTORIALISM

At this point, it might be illuminating to contrast holism with multifactorialism, the latter incorporating the idea that things have many causes, which, of course, they do. This notion has translated itself into a method in the 'alternative' medical field to give rise to a sort of eclecticism in practice. At the very least, it encourages the notion that 'causes' express themselves in discrete, parallel, 'linear' processes, evading or ignoring the fact that these processes are in reality entangled, requiring an approach that respects the 'mix'. Furthermore, the idea that for each dimension in which the patient's malfunction may manifest, there is a corresponding treatment modality, not only risks swamping the patient with too much treatment, it completely misses the point of the wisdom of holistic practice.

In relation to this notion, we have sometimes found that graduates of any one course in a therapeutic discipline have elected after a year or so in practice to supplement their knowledge with another course, e.g. the acupuncturist who takes up homeopathy; the osteopath who decides to do a little herbalism; the homeopath who embarks on a training in craniosacral therapy, or whatever. Now whereas this can have its value, there are caveats, and eclecticism and holism are very different things.

Anyway, as I often tell students, it takes a long time to become any good at *one* thing, and to retrain one's mind when it is only beginning to acquire facility and fluency in any one area of practice is not always wise. A discipline such as osteopathy, like any other, involves a commitment to a method, a conceptual framework, a 'language', a 'way of seeing', of processing data so that an effective treatment can be formulated or provided that is appropriate, skilful, precise and sufficient rather than excessive.

Secondly, holistic systems work with patterns in which 'causes' and context are entwined in an organic whole. If I can mix metaphors for a moment, this is 'sieved' through what we might call the 'osteopathic lens' so that the osteopathic method involves a specialised 'reading' of the patient to include presenting symptoms, clinical history, trauma history, mento-emotional habitus, personality and personal history, surgical and dental history, obstetric history, life-style factors etc. etc., and the interpretation of a 'structural matrix' of observable and palpable parameters that allow the osteopathic diagnosis to be formed. Sometimes this can be simple, almost linear; often it is not.

Now within this 'matrix' or pattern, there are priorities, one might say, points of emphasis. But the appreciation of its form involves the interlinking in the practitioner's mind of the ways in which the patient's 'story' is reflected in their structure and its expression in terms of motion, texture and the relationships between different structural elements in these terms. This can sound daunting but with skill and practice, the structural pattern is 'read' and the most suitable point(s) of contact, focus or point of 'entry' are discerned. So whereas the concept of 'holism' embraces the notion of interaction and the interconnectedness of the constituents of a system or organism, a holistic *approach* has to embody a way of influencing that system through the creation conceptually of a *pattern*. The characteristics of the pattern reflect the discipline in question and the way it is managed is based on a diagnostic and therapeutic set of methodological stages. These involve the product of observation and palpation entwined with clinical detail to form a diagnosis that is primarily 'osteopathic', in other words, in which the patient's habitus and history are reflected in the interplay of those 'structure/function bonds' that we looked at in Chapter 1, but which also enfolds a conventional clinical diagnosis that expands our understanding of the disease process while providing an element of safety in practice (which we look at in Chapter 11).

Part of what we 'read' is whether or not the various contextual parameters are relevant to the particular clinical situation and its demands, since they may not be in every instance. In other words, some findings might impact on the presenting problem to a limited degree or perhaps not at all.

How might it look?

Ultimately, we process the presenting information in an attempt to discern just how well it 'coheres'. It is the failure of such coherence that is reflected in a manually accessible pattern that contains dominant focal points or 'lesions' as we call them. Such lesions will be the structural reflections of changes in function that are acquired and accumulated from conception onwards and manifest, as described earlier, in altered 'mechanical' function. One hypothetical case might display all of the following. (Others are illustrated diagrammatically at the end of Chapter 4.)

- Intraosseous 'strain' and inertia at occipital condyle related to birth 'trauma'.
- Cranial membrane 'distortions' affecting temporal bone asymmetry and temporo-mandibular dysfunction, in turn reflecting in dental eruption and/ or occlusal problems.
- Scoliosis either inherited or predisposed to by the above.
- Intervertebral strain consequent on adaptive functional spinal patterns related to the above.
- Lumbo-sacral hypomobility or instability, with or without hip, psoas or piri-formis involvement as a reaction to trauma.
- Occupationally induced upper thoracic curve through long-term postural strain (often seen in violinists, hairdressers for example).
- Raised facilitation at points of particular strain in the intervertebral mechanism with or without somatico-visceral consequences.
- Postural alterations relating to the above but also reflecting a psycho-emotional attitude brought about in response to the sense of affliction that may or may not be created by the above.
- And finally, the product of the interplay of these various 'forces' that forms its own patterning and adaptive responses.

Depending on the approach, this complex patterning and its focal points will be interpreted accordingly. It is true that some patients will attend for help with one aspect of this complexity or one isolated symptom, and in some instances, the practitioner will 'extract' a causal ingredient (or structural corollary) that most directly gives expression to this or sustains it. But in truth, this approach might be limited if the other contextual ingredients are ignored with either short-lived benefit or even none at all. If the 'total lesion' is then to be considered, the various ingredients have to be interpreted so that, through a process of analysis and prioritising, a 'synthesis' can be reached that suggests a programme of treatment. It would clearly be unwise (and impossible) to 'manipulate' every aspect of this presenting picture; a strategy has to be formulated that is selective and specific and is based on criteria such as:

- Presenting symptoms: urgency, chronicity, 'irritability'/ 'volatility', degree of degeneration/pathology.
- History or 'order' of manifestation of structural features. (More recent 'layers' will often need to be addressed first in order to make more chronic layers amenable or 'available' to treatment).
- Complexity of the presenting pattern and the extent to which one's treatment has to be less 'direct', more oblique.
- Psycho-emotional significance of the pattern (either as cause or effect) again dictating a need to be more or less 'direct' in approach.

These along with many other clinical judgements help in the selection and implementation of an approach in which the *primary and secondary* nature of the ingredients of this 'total lesion' govern strategy.

(It is sometimes postulated that the 'cranial' model allows the body to prioritise and conduct this process for itself, but I would assert that even here, the practitioner is contacting the pattern with information and orientation that, as we'll look at later, 'loads' his or her contact so that observational and palpatory 'choices' are in fact made.)

On any one occasion, once these assessments become formulated into a 'pattern' *for that moment,* the theme, quality and *focus* of the treatment can be established, whichever treatment methods are favoured by the individual practitioner. With treatment, the pattern changes kaleidoscopically to be reassessed on each occasion as the process of reintegration unfolds. This elusive skill cannot be literally taught but the principles that make it possible can be instilled such that a 'relationship' with the material 'yields' the necessary diagnostic focus and treatment direction as a complex process of deduction based on the structure/function bonds and their interplay as described in the first chapter.

THE IMPORTANCE OF PATTERN

It is *pattern,* then, that is 'greater than the sum of the parts'. It is the product of interaction, but such interaction can be highly complex, sometimes even imponderable. The holistic model can, however, make this imponderable accessible. In fact, there may be no other way to get near it.

As outlined in the last chapter, it is 'motion patterns' that primarily concern the osteopath as the continuum on which we examine and assess relative function, and though these manifestations of altered mobility take different forms and reveal different qualities, we begin to 'read' the patient's body in a functional sense through these patterns of mobility along with the textural, circulatory and neural features that inevitably accompany them. Whilst the altered motion characteristics of particular structures are important – and these have formed the basis of osteopathic thinking thanks to contributors such as Fryette (1954) with the functional motion characteristics of vertebrae – it is the integrated motion of the spine and body structure as a whole that is more revealing and relevant to changes in physiology. The formation in the practitioner's mind of a working 'pattern' based on these findings is key to an osteopathic diagnosis, a diagnosis which enfolds a conventional medical appraisal whilst being bonded firmly to the patient's clinical, personal and historical details. It is virtually axiomatic that the patient's 'story' *has* to be reflected in their tissues; it is our responsibility to read it as accurately as possible and to develop an appropriate therapeutic strategy. Some simple examples of these 'lesion patterns' as we call them are considered in the next chapter. They help to prioritise our findings in order to construct the treatment strategy. But for the moment, let it be emphasised that the patterns and processes that we address in treatment – the ones that sustain and express the patient's symptoms – might reflect entirely different symptoms in another patient or none at all in another. These patterns, in other words, represent a window through which we contact a 'dynamic' that is unique. In this way we work with 'cause' in an entirely different way from the more reductionist disciplines of orthodoxy. Without the complex context that characterises the individual patient, the isolated lesion is almost meaningless.

HOLISTIC TECHNIQUE

Osteopathy, like many other disciplines, has developed techniques and procedures that are specifically geared to the achieving of certain effects. Some of these encourage 'pumping' effects of circulating fluids, e.g. drainage techniques. Others are locally applied mobilising techniques applied to bony and soft tissues: joints, muscle, fascia, etc. Many of these are subtle 'release' procedures as in balanced ligamentous and membranous tension, 'functional' technique, and 'muscle energy technique' (MET). Some techniques are designed to create an inhibitory or sedative effect on tissue and particularly on neuromuscular function. And it has to be said that many of these locally applied procedures are highly effective, achieving not only local improvements but also 'whole-body' benefits. Some of these treatments are designed to counter specifically identified problems as in the effects of trauma.

However, it should be remembered that the body's response (even in trauma), is systemic and is organised or patterned around the localised 'trigger' phenomenon or lesion. For example, the tension and congestion at the thoracic outlet that predispose to sinus infection or congestive headache are anatomically and physiologically complex. Furthermore, this phenomenon rarely exists in isolation but is part of a body-wide pattern that helps to sustain the problem, so that treatments that are merely local in conception might be doomed to fail or to have short-term benefits.

So when we read of the inspired techniques developed by Still, Sutherland and countless other exponents over the years, it is useful to remember that they will not usually have been conceived in isolation of the matrix of 'whole body' patterning that forms their proper context. A lesion may give rise to an effect that is considered dominant in the production of a symptom or of malfunction, but its context in a holistic sense is every bit as important clinically and therapeutically.

The osteopathic lens

As I've said, all holistic systems would subscribe to the complex interlocking of the many functional elements that comprise human bodies and human beings. The osteopathic 'view' of this totality is defined as it is brought into focus by a perceptual and conceptual orientation. This, in turn, is the product of certain observational and palpatory skills coupled with the aforementioned concepts that link 'structure' and 'function'. This 'lens' makes certain information available into which we, as practitioners, delve in order to select, to question, to synthesise and to deduce; and a diagnosis emerges that couples with conventional medical theory to form a safe and responsible clinical approach. However, this 'conventional' part supports but does not generate osteopathic diagnosis. It valuably interlinks biological and pathophysiological detail but cannot, of itself, provide the necessary framework that elicits the osteopathic treatment strategy. For that, many of the other features outlined in this book have to play their part. Meanwhile, the osteopathic lens is both a perceptual and conceptual 'device' without which the osteopathic method would cease to be.

While it is accessed through an appreciation of the 'strands' that link structure and function, there has been a tendency to 'over-segmentalise' the approach in manipulative disciplines, usually along the lines of what connects the anatomy to the symptom via neural and circulatory pathways in a somewhat linear fashion. However, most clinical problems are a composite of several mechanisms, each of which is reflected in structure and which are bound together through the body's mechanical reciprocity of function. So the orchestrated reciprocity of body systems is most vitally complemented by the integrated operation of the structure itself. The overarching approach born of holism is the only way to access this satisfactorily. Some achieve this through a 'whole body' approach enshrined in the 'general osteopathic treatment' of 'body adjustment' as it is called. Others pursue an equally holistic method via a conception of the whole body pattern that enfolds points of maximum mechanical, physiological and 'energetic' potency or relevance. Specific and strategic treatment of these 'points' produces a staged resolution of the pattern with the body's own highly orchestrated responses stimulated maximally. Such specificity can be exercised to varying degrees and through different technical methods depending on practitioner orientation and preferences as well as the demands of the patient's system, symptoms, typology, etc.

CONCLUSION

The application of holistic paradigms requires the implementation of models. The function of most complex things, especially human beings, is the expression of so many interlocking variables that it is inconceivable that we can know them all, and a change in just one detail can alter the complex patterning of the whole. So we need an overarching principle, a model, by which to negotiate this complexity. Reductionist methods are wonderful for examining detail; but 'things happen', unpredictable variables insinuate themselves into our lives, and life is expressed where multiple factors coalesce; a model helps us interpret just *how* this process expresses itself in both health and disease. This 'coalescence' is not always reducible to known elements, just as reality and experience are not dependent upon explanation and analysis: gravity, after all, existed before Newton!

REFERENCES

Abramson, J, 2005, *Overdosed America*, Harper Perennial.
Fryette, HH, 1954, *The Principles of Osteopathic Technique*, Academy of Applied Osteopathy.
Goswami, A, 1993, *The Self-Aware Universe*, Putnam Penguin (1995).
Heisenberg, W, 1958, *Physics and Philosophy*, Harper Torchbooks.
Helman, C, 2006, *Suburban Shaman*, Hammersmith.
Ingber, D, 1998, The architecture of life, *Scientific American* 278(1):48–57.
Pienta, K J & Coffey, D S, 1991, Cellular harmonic information transfer through a tissue tensegrity-matrix system, *Medical Hypotheses* 34:88–95.
Pischinger, A, 2007, *The Extracellular Matrix and Ground Regulation*, North Atlantic Books.

Chapter 4

Reciprocity, Relationship, Spaces

M any years ago, I participated in a study group, in Maine, USA. A group of like-minded people from the profession on both sides of the Atlantic had been selected, ostensibly to share their thoughts and ideas on the practice of the osteopathic art, more especially in the 'cranial' field.

Our brief was for each of us to put together a short lecture that said something about our deepest thoughts, ideas, even problems in the execution of this wonderfully complex yet subtle end of the osteopathic continuum. We were asked to be candid, uninhibited even, for we were looking potentially at areas of doubt, wonder and even uncertainty, in a group of quite seasoned practitioners.

Some reinterpreted this brief and gave instead informative vignettes on aspects of our work and some of its physiological ramifications. Others were of a more soul-baring mentality and spoke bravely of the deeper challenges and vulnerabilities that assail practitioners in our field.

I suppose I struck some sort of middle ground and started on a theme that truly grasped my imagination and continues to do so to this day. A few years later when the same, slightly enlarged group gathered again on this side of the Atlantic, in Cornwall in fact, and we were invited to do more of the same, I found myself voicing a similar theme and this material has continued to be part of my undergraduate lectures ever since. The group was known as The Old England New England Study Group and had been largely inspired by James Jealous DO, one of our profession's truly fine minds.

My talk on both occasions opened with a bit of an 'act', as the essential introvert gave vent to his inner performer. However, I sought to offer a visual image that I called the 'doughnut', inspired by the distant memory of a ditty quoted by a psychiatrist/entertainer (if that's not a contradiction in terms) on a record that my parents owned and that I remembered hearing when I was about 12 years old. The humorist was a psychiatrist called Dr Murray Banks who had presumably opted for a lighter way of making a living, and the ditty went:

'As you travel on through life, my friend, whatever be your goal
Keep your eye upon the doughnut and not upon the hole.'

In psychotherapeutic terms, this was a serious if simple point extolling the virtues of positive thought: focus on what matters in life, not on the dross.

In my little presentation, meanwhile, I wanted to make the case for 'the hole', and I wanted to do it for two reasons, both to do with 'reciprocity, relationship and space', not dross, and despite the rather facetious nature of this prologue, this issue sits at the heart of the osteopathic concept for me and, like much of my material, involves the 'wider world'. So let's look at the importance of *interplay* and *pattern* and their relevance to our work.

INTERPLAY

One of the fundamental tenets of osteopathy, as well as other systems of health care, is the importance of the interactivity of body systems. This interactivity means that, subject to degrees of adaptability, disturbances in one system *potentially* (not inevitably), produce malfunction in other systems. This may seem self-evident, i.e. that the neuro-hormonal system, for example, impacts on the digestive system which in turn impacts on the renal and biliary systems etc. etc. But the notion of reciprocal functioning of these systems in relation to the musculoskeletal or structural system seems to elude many people both medical and otherwise. Conventionally, our analytical approach has thrived on separation, specialisation and analysis rather than synthesis. Meanwhile, the interactive nature of 'structure' (the musculoskeletal and connective tissue systems) and 'function' (visceral function and physiology) is the central axiom of the osteopathic credo.

There are many respects in which the concept of reciprocity expresses itself in the arena of psycho-physical function and therapeutics:

1. Organisms operate in a system of interplay with the wider environment, their immediate surroundings, geographical location, climate, local agriculture and broader ecosystem.
2. They also respond in an interactive fashion with other living systems in a variety of structured ways depending on their relationship with these systems (biological, symbiotic, social, economic, familial, intimate/emotional, etc.)
3. The so-called biological systems within any one organism are in a state of functional reciprocity, i.e. they are interdependent.
4. The structural elements of the body are themselves in a state of functional reciprocity in that the organism functions as a dynamic whole and what happens in any one area is reflected throughout the whole. No single part of the body has a functional significance that is independent and discreet. Its significance and operation are dependent and interactive with its context.
5. Interpersonal relationships affect the above, and strategic interpersonal relationships such as the patient/practitioner relationship are a special type of interaction subject to specific rules that provide a template by which a unique 'dance' is subject to particular protocols.

The concept of interactivity implies interplay and a mechanism or mechanisms by which this interplay should take place. We might examine some of the processes involved and the theories behind them. But to begin, I'd like to refer to another of my illustrative digressions, based on another of my little obsessions: pots.

Pots

A long-standing interest in contemporary ceramics began in around the mid 1970s, and a modest beginning as a collector involved the acquisition of a book by Bernard Leach, the forefather of modern ceramicists in this country. In it, a phrase about the magic of form, the interplay of the foot of a bowl with its lip, and the way that this relationship or juxtaposition is modulated by the quality of the glaze, has been an inspiration as well as an influence. The tension, emotional power, energetic power and communication and hence the experience for the observer are totally dependent on the artist's power to harness these relationships for the expression of an idea, emotion or creative purpose. And the conceptual or notional 'space' between these qualities is a 'plenum', full of information, a 'glue' loaded with the power that harnesses the potential or the meaning of the piece. Without these loaded spaces, there is no context, relationship or whole; the individual ingredients are sterile, inert and insignificant.

In the case of pots, this creates a quality that we can loosely describe as beauty; the communication of something that is transcendent in its properties of wholeness, a wholeness that – as the cliché goes – is greater than the sum of its parts.

As I said, the beauty of these objects began to make an impact on me back in the mid 1970s when the quieter moments in a practice waiting to build were spent perusing beautiful things in Marylebone in London where one would be tempted to spend money one hadn't yet earned.

One such haven of temptation was a gallery selling many beautiful craft objects including fine ceramics. The seduction began as I responded to these wonderful forms and persuaded myself of ways to divert portions of my meagre income to invest in some of these. It also led me to meet Lucie Rie, an inspirational woman and one of the greatest ceramicists of the 20th century.

The habit of holidaying in the West Country took me to a part of England that had hosted many artists, painters and ceramicists – most notably Bernard Leach himself and his potting dynasty – so the obsession could also be continued and indulged on holiday, without interruption! On one such trip, I came across that book by Bernard Leach called *The Potter's Challenge* and read with the fascination that often accompanies a resonance with something fundamental in one's own field: the familiar idea of the integrity and the 'meaning' conveyed in the pot that derives from its intrinsic dynamics; the interplay of its features, their interface, its wholeness (Leach, 1975).

The movement and the life generated by this interplay is what can give a pot its aesthetic value, and I warmly recall an occasion when, on one of my visits to David Leach's pottery (Bernard's son), I was to choose between two simple, beautiful bowls to add to my small collection. David tried to help me in my dilemma and pointed out that one was 'more perfect' while the other was the better pot. Well, in those naïve days, that simply didn't help much so I bought the 'perfect' one and only later, in coming to understand what he meant, learned why the other pot was the better piece. It was the lack of clean perfection in the latter piece that revealed its 'tension' and in that quality, it conveyed more movement, more life. The tension created by relative 'motion', relative form – not to mention their interaction with glaze and colour – was the *life* in the piece and the joy it gave the observer. For me, the pots by Lucie Rie exemplify this almost more than the work of any other potter.

When it comes to aesthetics, it is, of course, quite usual, if unnecessary, to ascribe our responses to works of beauty or of art to this 'juxtaposition' or interplay of different qualities or characteristics. Quite often, we are even aware that our responses to one another and the power of attraction are based on the interplay of different features of appearance, personality and mannerism. But when considering hard fact and information, an analytical process takes over and we work with the conviction that, to know more, we must dissect. Whereas this is true to a point, it is ultimately impossible to understand something if it is only assessed in terms of its parts without appraising the effect of the interplay of those parts. Werner Heisenberg was not only speaking of sub-atomic particles when he said that something has significance only in terms of its relationship to something else. And distinguished physicist Henry Stapp writes: '*the physical world is . . . not a structure built out of independently existing unanalyzable entities, but rather a web of relationships between elements whose meanings arise wholly from their relationships to the whole.*' (Stapp, 1971)

In science, many concepts such as this – the concept of interconnectedness – have been extrapolated from quantum theory and we are constantly being cautioned about transposing the concepts spawned by quantum theory and applying them simplistically to the 'macro' world. However, as Richard Feynman states, 'quantum theory is just about the best theory we have about just about everything.' The quantum/Newtonian dichotomy relates to our way of perceiving things as well as their underlying nature. And the assertion that the relevance and meaning of something are related to its interactions within its context – we shall expand on 'context' later – is, I feel, fundamental to our relationship with our world. *In osteopathy, it is at the core of the whole approach and absolutely basic to an effective mode of practice.*

William Sutherland entreated his students to look at the 'spaces' between anatomical planes of fascia, between structures; the place where 'relationship' resides. The first time I heard Sutherland quoted in this context was in a lecture by Dr Anne Wales, one of Sutherland's pupils and a life-long exponent of the osteopathic art. It bonded magically with Bernard Leach and the pots, the fascination with interplay and the mystery of the information held in the 'space', in the relationship between parts.

Adding to this, I soon began yanking into my consciousness, the earliest seeds of my struggle with quantum theory and the long, slow and troubling journey to look at energetic expression and transfer, and slowly I began to absorb those ideas about the ways that information travelled through the body other than through neural, neuro-hormonal and circulatory pathways.

Interplay in structure

But before looking at some of those, I want to dwell on something absolutely fundamental to the practice of osteopathy and that is the interdependence and functional interplay of the various structural elements themselves: the bones, joints, muscles, tendons, ligaments and fascia, the last of which will give us much to consider in the light of cutting edge science and serving to confirm the huge importance given to fascia by Still over 100 years ago.

One misconception held by many patients is that they feel a problem or a pain that they sense as 'muscular' suggests the need for massage; rather than the 'bone' or' joint' problem that makes it a case for the osteopath. It would be unreasonable to expect patients to make considered judgements about such matters as the functional interplay between the various structural elements of the body only really starts to come to life when it is examined anatomically and physiologically. It has, therefore, to be emphasised that muscles, bones, joints, tendons etc. comprise a unit of function such that joint problems, for example, rarely exist in isolation; related tissues of all kinds are of necessity involved, even those that would *appear* to be functionally separate. There is often, therefore, no simple prescription for one type of therapy over another based on the locus of the symptom or the tissue type involved.

One intriguing example of just how 'strange' the interplay of structural elements can be involves a resistant case brought to me some years ago for a second opinion in which the patient suffered acute abdominal and lower back pain that had resisted all attempts at treatment. We finally analysed the 'strain pattern' giving rise to diaphragmatic and psoas over-contraction as centred on a membranous strain in the intracranial mechanism, itself secondary to a restriction (or lesion) at one of the palatines, disturbing the spheno-maxillary relationship. This in turn was secondary to recent dental extraction that coincided with the onset of the symptom.

Structure governs structure

Students of osteopathy have struggled for decades with the issue of what we sometimes call the 'spinal mechanics' and we'll look at that subject in a moment. However, the whole point about this struggle is to find a means of embracing a model that allows us to circumnavigate the complex web of interaction of the thousands of structural elements that comprise the body so that a therapeutic strategy can be formed. In other words, how can we interpret the structural make-up of the individual patient in a way that makes 'mechanical' sense?

Moving on from the osteopathic axiom that 'structure and function are interdependent', we have then to consider just how 'structure governs structure' as well; and while it is undoubtedly true that each patient is an individual and that patients all have their ways of coping, adapting and compensating, it is still possible to determine principles and rules by which to map the patient's musculoskeletal pattern and to marry it to the patient's story, their history and presenting clinical picture, not to mention aspects of their mento-emotional profile. Whilst observing these patterns, it is useful to remember that any given structural pattern will express itself in an individuated, if not entirely unique, way. In this sense, it becomes futile to expect a particular somatic 'lesion' or pattern to produce the same symptom picture in every patient (although there may be ingredients that have predictable effects), and as we know, many somatic dysfunctions exist in patients without any symptoms at all, so well are they compensated or managed by an otherwise healthy constitution. At the same time, this quiescent scenario can be deceptive as asymptomatic structural dysfunctions can be part of long-term predispositions that can erupt later, and herein lies the importance of conservative prophylaxis.

PATTERN

At the outset, let me say that the structural patterns I wish to illustrate at the end of this section are not so much causative as reflective of the complex interacting processes that, in all of us, express something of our *inner being*, the 'who we are', along with our coping and our struggles, some of which result in a failure of good health, however slight or however profound. In this way, our structural personae *are* our health records. Where they *are* causative, they are often the result of trauma, patterns of body 'use', or of genetically acquired or congenital abnormalities. In other cases, elements that we may consider to be *primarily* causal are entirely likely to be 'non-structural', for example, psycho-emotional, circumstantial, biochemical, viral, toxic, pathological, etc. However, it is the way that 'structure' renders these influences accessible therapeutically that is important to us. We evolved these patterns themselves as a way of demonstrating the interaction of the many pertinent ingredients in the patient's presenting 'picture' but more especially to prioritise these factors in order to give the osteopathic analysis or diagnosis 'shape' and to develop an effective treatment strategy that avoids any superfluous or unnecessary intervention. As such, this endeavour grew partly out of the SAT model but as a principle, was very much aligned with Rollin Becker's 'cranial' model. Whereas from Becker's perspective, the structural pattern would be conceived in bioenergetic terms and largely manifest in the connective tissue with an 'energetic' focus (the 'eye' of the storm), the SAT model would impute a 'primary' focus of dysfunction, usually (though not always) centred on a vertebral segment and its related tissues, reflexes and dynamics; in other words, 'a spinal lesion'. This notion of a 'primary' can itself be divided into two: the first representing this focal point of structural dysfunction at any given moment; the second being the most significant somatic dysfunction historically, usually of traumatic origin and viewed diagnostically as the force behind the various compensatory and adaptive 'secondary' lesions that complete the matrix of dysfunction, with their layers of physiological effects. In my own terminology, I would refer to these in lectures as 'focal' and 'base' primaries respectively to distinguish between them.

PATTERN EVALUATION

Structural patterns are evaluated not only in terms of anatomical balance or gross structural appearance; they are more importantly assessed in terms of mobility, subtle motility and texture as well as, 'energetic' patterns and dynamics that are so much a part of osteopathy in the 'cranial' field, a subject to be discussed later. But whichever approach is espoused, the concept of mechanical functional unity is paramount such that without it, treatment can become shallow, too regional, unconstitutional and frequently ineffectual or temporary in its usefulness.

It's not all in the mind; it's not all in the spine either

At this point, it may be helpful to clear up one of the many misconceptions about this work. It is sometimes thought that because osteopaths treat many patients with a variety of ills through the body framework or structure, they presumably contend that all such ills are *caused* by malfunctions *in* the structure. This is to misinterpret the fundamental concept of holism and reciprocity. The integral role of 'structure' with all other aspects of 'function', as outlined above, makes structure a perfect point of access in the treatment of all systems – whether or not the initiating or trigger factor resides in the musculoskeletal system, which of course it frequently does not.

The obsession with what I can only call a culturally instilled 'linearity' would have us believe that most things are caused by a dominant factor that we call 'cause' that functions, if not in isolation, then by dominating all other factors in a one-way process of cause and effect. Much scientific and medical endeavour is spent on isolating these 'causes' to the exclusion of other factors in order to prove their causative dominance and to fashion treatments that 'fit' them. (A perennial example of this assertion of dominance is the *nature/ nurture* debate: the fight to assert the primacy of genes over environment, in its broadest sense, or vice versa).

It is not merely the influence of 'systems' thinking and quantum theory that tell us what common sense told us long before, that things are usually the manifestation of multiple causes and their interactions. For example, toxic levels of industrial pollutants may be maintained below danger levels, but what happens when several sub-threshold pollutants combine in the atmosphere or the water supply? Does the product of their interaction remain at safe levels? Gradually, the significance of this type of phenomenon is percolating current thinking and policymaking in some departments, but it's taken a while.

Now there are, of course, examples of the primacy of certain causative factors. Perhaps 2% of disease is caused by an abnormal gene. Some virulent infections are certainly triggered by definitive causative agents – viruses, bacteria, etc. – but even here, it can be said that illness manifests as a product of the interaction of these causes with a susceptible constitution and a weakened immunity. The embryologist Erich Blechschmidt emphasised the importance of external influences on the developing embryo stating that genetic activity is reactive as well as proactive and that *mechanical forces outside of or on the surface of the developing embryo can direct the course of the development of the embryo with as much certainty as genes or metabolism* (Blechschmidt, 1978).

So, notwithstanding the primacy of *some* causes, health is about adaptability, resilience and constitutional integrity. Causal primacy is evidenced in such things as toxicity, e.g. septic foci, heavy metals including dental amalgams and particularly virulent micro-organisms, especially those to which the patient has not built up a resistance (encountered through travel, for example), trauma, *alongside* genetic and constitutional predispositions.

Let it be said at this point that the concept of interconnectedness, of reciprocity of function, is not anathema to conventional medical theorists. It is simply that so often, the therapeutic approach that is implemented is extremely targeted and linear, and in this sense, the body is not always treated with respect to its orchestrated unity.

But back to osteopathy. It is the fortunate interplay of the body's systems in a complex web of interaction that allows the osteopath (as well as other physical therapeutic systems) to access the potential that draws on the powerful process of self-correction. Indeed, so often, prime causes *do* exist in structure, and we'll look at examples of these below, but clearly they don't *have* to exist for a case to be accessible through osteopathic treatment. The saying (even by some osteopaths themselves) that a case is 'osteopathic' to the extent to which the cause is in the musculoskeletal system is not merely misleading; it is wrong! The injection of the osteopathic method into the complex interactive matrix of the body's physiology is not only possible, it is highly effective. However, primary causes can and often do reside in the musculoskeletal system whether they produce symptoms in the body frame-work e.g. the bread-and-butter cases of many osteopaths: back pain, extremity pain, headache etc. etc., or symptoms anywhere else: in virtually any of the organ systems. Most of these are treatable where they represent abnormalities of function (i.e. they are 'functional' complaints) though there may be pathology present to some degree. However, where pathological factors over-ride as they do in perhaps 15–20% of cases, osteopathy might be limited, inappropriate or simply useless. The responsible clinician has to make this judgement as immediate referral might be essential, even life-saving.

At this juncture, it may be worth tackling a popular contention about the advantages of so-called 'natural therapeutics' methods in respect of causes. It has often been said that the prime value of these therapies is that they treat causes and not effects. This is such an oversimplification that it needs to be contested which I hope the foregoing manages to achieve. Clearly, causes are frequently so profound, inaccessible or irreversible that, despite their impor-tance, they cannot always be tackled.

Secondly, if we truly hold to the 'holographic' notion of body function, we can subscribe to the efficacy of a treatment that reduces the severity of the patient's response to 'cause', enhancing their ability to cope, reducing the 'input' of symptom, pain or other abnormal neural input, all of which make the condition self-perpetuating and deleterious to the constitution.

Though natural methods might well be preferred, simple analgesics and other medications, prescribed short-term, buy the patient time and resilience too, allowing the natural tendency for homoeostasis to establish itself. In this way, all effective treatments can buy this advantage. Palliation has its place, provided the cost (with medication) is not too great in terms of toxicity or risk. However, even then it may, of course, be the only expedient to consider.

PALLIATION

Many osteopathic procedures have powerful and direct effects that are inci-dental to the complex interactive mechanisms I have been describing. These are often focussed on palliative pain relief in bony and soft tissues, the relief of soft tissue and connective tissue tensions and their effects on blood vessels, lymph channels and organs themselves, and direct drainage techniques, e.g.

the various lymphatic pump techniques and sinus drainage procedures. (There are many equivalents of these in other disciplines, e.g. physiotherapy.)

Functional reciprocity

The functional unity of the body structure, being central to osteopathic practice, necessitates a model or system by which we can access it therapeutically. In an almost crude, simplistic and ultimately clumsy way, some practitioners of manipulative treatment have taken the 'more the merrier' approach to treatment and kneaded and manipulated everything they could get their hands on. This 'approach' to unity is not only haphazard but can set up so many interference patterns of response in the body that temporary palliation is the result at best, turbulence, overstimulation and irritation, at worst.

So intelligent models have been created that not only explain the nature of the body's mechanical interactivity, they also make possible a therapeutic approach or strategy that assists the body in making its own therapeutic responses, ideally with minimal intervention or interference.

SPINAL MECHANICS

Students of osteopathy have struggled with models of spinal mechanics as long as they have existed. But for all their shortcomings, they have been invaluable in helping us negotiate the mechanisms of musculoskeletal function and malfunction that have allowed the creation of treatment strategies and protocols. Above all, they have emphasised and illustrated the unity of function of the body structure and have helped explain why things happen in the body structure the way they do.

There are really three dominant systems of 'mechanics' that we osteopaths live with that have underpinned our diagnostic and treatment models. The first which is termed 'the spinal mechanics' is the notion promulgated by J.M. Littlejohn (1956), later elaborated by T.E. Hall (1956) and John Wernham (1956), complete with its 'curves, arches and pivots'. The second is the model of 'reciprocal tension' that sits at the heart of the IVM or 'cranial' approach. And the third is the 'tensegrity' model, originally pioneered and based on the concept by the architect Buckminster Fuller and later adapted and applied to the sphere of anatomy by Stephen Levin and Donald Ingber. All three models promote the same message: that structural function is an holistic phenomenon in which the parts are in a state of interaction and interconnectedness. Many vitally useful functional patterns have been extrapolated from these and are used every day by many if not all exponents of the osteopathic art.

As this is not a textbook, it is the implication of all this as a principle of good practice that is my point rather than a thorough exposition of each system. For that, I refer the reader to the excellent *Osteopathy* by Parsons & Marcer (2006) where these concepts are explained analytically and where typological concepts as elucidated by Goldthwaite (1866-1961), Sheldon (1898-1977), Kretchmer (1888-1964), Dummer and others show how differing body types reflect different susceptibilities clinically and call for different 'styles' of intervention therapeutically.

But briefly, we'll take the 'spinal mechanics' model first. This was developed by John Martin Littlejohn (1865-1947) who not only influenced osteopathic thinking by expanding its physiological relevance, but elaborated a system of biomechanics based on the balanced function of the arches and curves in the spine and the designation of certain vertebral segments as pivots and keystones within this mechanical model. This, like many other concepts within osteopathy, was a sincere attempt to develop a schema that produced a workable model that gave diagnosis and treatment a methodological basis. Its impact on practice has, for many within the profession, been quite profound, though for others it has been seen as too static. But its value is greater if its principles are interpreted with flexibility and its tenets are not too rigidly applied.

The essential message of any model of spinal mechanics is the demonstration of reciprocal function: the interactivity of different spinal regions and different vertebral segments such that both a diagnostic appraisal and a therapeutic strategy can be accurately formulated provided that the diagnostic assessment serves as a template that can be tailored to serve the individual patient.

When we look at the reciprocal tension membrane as a concept within the 'cranial' approach, we find a similar 'dogmatic trap' in which the concept implies a mechanical link within the dural mechanism that would intimate a physical connection between occiput and sacrum in which the dura performed as a type of pulley. This is to misinterpret the process by which informational (and tensional) transfer is conducted throughout the body. In both examples, we see a need to impute a graphic and over-mechanical process, both of which compromise reality for the sake of intellectual accessibility. However, for all their shortcomings, they both underscore a principle that is invaluable in practice, and like most rules, they need to be assimilated before the right to break them is earned.

TENSEGRITY

This interactive concept was broadened with the application of the concept of 'tensegrity' to the body; a concept with its origins in architecture and the theories of Buckminster Fuller. The tensegrous function of the connective tissue totally energises the osteopathic concept. Its complex meshwork of interrelated bioelectrically charged strands operating through a balance of tension and compression contains both the mechanism that regulates the body as a structure as well as a matrix that both influences and responds to physiology. It is as if the functional operation of the body is expressed and organised in this mechanical matrix, 'function'revealing itself as 'structure'; 'function' *being* 'structure' and vice versa.

Donald Ingber is the cell biologist who has contributed enormously to the understanding of this phenomenon in which the mechanics of structural function are yoked to the biological and physiological control of organisms:

> '. . . the mechanical properties, behaviour and movement of our bodies, are as important for human health as chemicals and genes. However, only recently have scientists and physicians begun to appreciate the key role which mechanical forces play in biological control at the molecular and cellular levels.'
>
> (Ingber, 2008)

In referring to Ingber's contribution, Mae-Wan Ho (2008) elaborates his notion that '*the whole cell and its "solid state" of membrane skeleton, cytoskeleton, microtrabecular lattice and nuclear scaffold, form an interconnected "tensegrity" system that always deforms or changes as a whole when local stresses and strains are experienced.*'

Ho recalls the birth of the tensegrity concept and its originator, architect and polymath, Buckminster Fuller who described this concept of *tensional integrity* as a structural system based on the dynamic interaction of discontinuous compression elements connected by continuous tension cables. Ingber (2008) and others (Levin, 1982) have shown how this concept is reflected in the entire organism '*with emphasis on the extracellular matrix in mechanically coupling cells to coordinate and control their structure and function . . .*' (Ho, 2008)

A principle of this nature that underpins the view of the body structure as an integrated whole whilst, at the same time, expanding on its role in the physiological regulation and control of the organism, is a gift to osteopathy that validates its essential model.

The concepts of the spinal mechanics, tensegrity and the reciprocal tension ingredient of the 'cranial' approach that we look at in the next chapter, are all powerful models by which we can explore and work with the important phenomenon of interactivity and functional reciprocity without which the osteopathic concept would itself be infinitely poorer. Without them, we would struggle to work with the complex nature of pain and illness through the diligent manual approach that characterises the osteopathic art.

While the potential for reciprocal function to express itself through the body is almost infinite in its variability, especially throughout the connective tissue matrix, there are certain themes that present frequently and there are typical structural patterns on to which a corrective strategy can be superimposed.

Here then (see Figures 1-15) are some examples of such cranio-spinal patterns that reflect structural interactions, the priorities on which we might focus in terms of 'primary' and 'secondary' lesions in the spine and craniosacral mechanism, and potential consequences for the hypothetical patient. They demonstrate some of the principles we employ in osteopathic diagnosis.

These patterns are not, of course, definitive. They are examples of the way that the dominant structural changes may combine to reflect the patient's clinical picture. Above all, they are illustrative of the functional interplay and reciprocity in our patients and the way that the mechanism of symptom production can be enfolded in these patterns, patterns in which that mechanism might appear physically remote from the primary musculoskeletal factor or 'lesion'. Diagrammatically, they reflect the dominant areas of dysfunction in the osteopathic sense in each hypothesised pattern, displaying regions of altered mobility, tissue texture, stability, irritability and energetic quality. Naturally, individual patients will present specific details interwoven into these patterns which will modulate both diagnosis and prescribed treatment.

Many of these hypothetical patterns are best suited to the 'structural' perspective since, within the connective tissue matrix and the Involuntary Mechanism (IVM), focal points of inertia or strain can be almost anywhere, distorting the whole body matrix in totally idiosyncratic ways, or producing generalised and system-wide qualities such as hyperflexion, hyperextension, torsion, etc. Such distortions can, of course, be entwined in the patterns below and ideally the practitioner is alive to this. Nevertheless, certain of these examples show an inevitable interplay between 'structural' and IVM diagnostic criteria. Above all, remember that these examples are typical, not definitive, but demonstrate principles we employ in practice all the time.

Note, the 'lesion' areas that we would designate as *primary,* or perhaps of major *causal* significance are highlighted in **bold.**

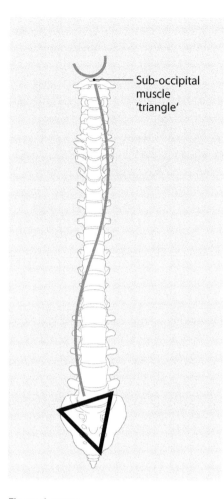

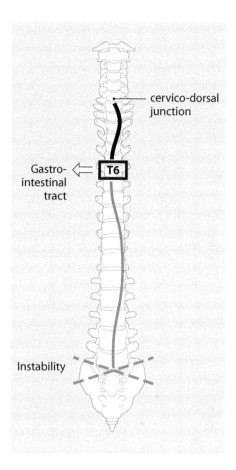

Figure 1 notes

Simple 'linear' reciprocity where the spinal mechanics reflect compensatory patterns. A lower back (lumbo-sacral or sacro-iliac) 'primary' producing compensatory curves through lumbar, thoracic and cervical regions with resulting tension centred in the sub-occipital muscle 'triangle' triggering headache. The site of the 'primary' might be asymptomatic: a principle central to osteopathic thinking, that the symptom is not necessarily a guide to the locus sustaining the 'primary' lesion.

Figure 2 notes

The upper thoracic 'short lateral curve' – a common feature of postural habits, often occupational. As a 'primary', it leads here to secondary dysfunctions destabilizing the cervico-dorsal junction, irritating the mid-thoracic intervertebral units with raised facilitation and possible somatico-visceral consequences (gastro-intestinally, via the mid-thoracic sympathetic chain). A compensatory disequilibrium at the lumbo-sacral junction often renders it unstable which can be as likely to produce some lower back and lower extremity syndromes as if the 'primary' were in the lumbo-sacral spine itself.

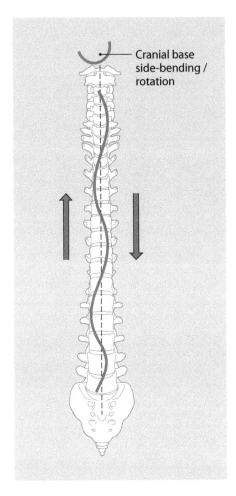

Cranial base side-bending / rotation

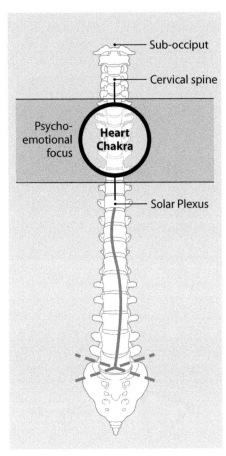

Sub-occiput

Cervical spine

Psycho-emotional focus

Heart Chakra

Solar Plexus

Figure 3 notes

Complex thoraco-lumbar curves can be resistant to structural treatment where connective tissue or fascial strain patterns dominate the picture as here with a shear in the sagittal plain extending throughout the body and reflected (and often diag-nosed) at the cranial base as a sphe-nobasilar 'side-bending/rotation strain'.

Figure 4 notes

The pooling of emotional energy targeting the upper thorax and 'heart centre' (or chakra) can not only produce palpable changes in the upper thoracic fascia (with its own dynamic effects), but can also result in somatic changes at the upper thoracic intervertebral segments. Associated stress can have similar effects in the lower thorax and solar (celiac) plexus, with fear, anxiety, anger and other reactions focusing here. Chronic patterns of this nature disturb both neck and lower body mechanics with possible sequelae in these areas, e.g. pain, dysfunction or degenerative change.

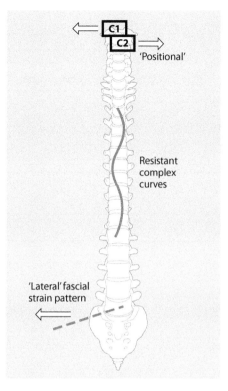

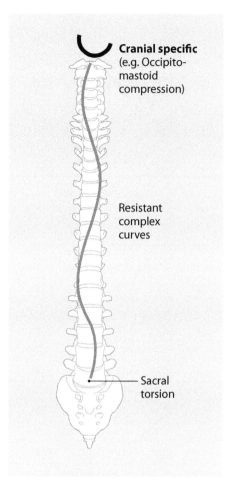

Figure 5a notes

The 'positional lesion', reflected in SAT diagnostic theory, can dominate the structural pattern so significantly that treatment approaches that do not address it can be ineffective. The connective tissue strain patterns might be eccentric with, for example, a series of 'transverse shears' throughout the body reflecting a *lateral* component in the lesion complex at C1/2 or C2/3 along with possible rotational, latero-flexed, hypo- or hyper-flexion elements. Whatever the configuration, when the lesion reflects a mal-relationship beyond the normal physiological ranges of motion, such 'positional' lesions can be overwhelming both mechanically and physiologically, requiring manipulation that precisely respects the detail of the intervertebral relationship.

Figure 5b notes

Specific intracranial, interosseous and intraosseous compressions might have similar consequences to the 'positional' example in 5a.

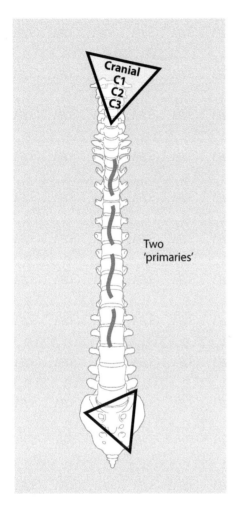

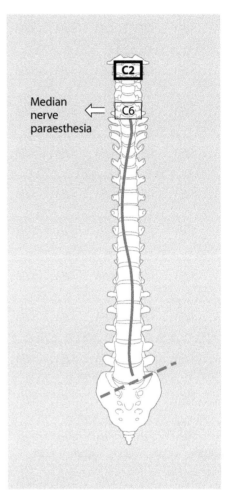

Figure 6 notes

Dominant musculoskeletal lesions can be sustained at different periods in a patient's life, each having powerful effects on the body structure as a whole and each with its compensatory 'layers'. Naturally these layers do not remain discrete but compound one another to produce complex changes to motion patterns throughout the spine. In practice, the more recent 'layer' should be addressed first.

Figure 7 notes:

Certain lesions can dominate the spinal picture powerfully. Secondary lesion states might generate the patient's symptom picture directly along clear nerve pathways as here with median nerve paraesthesiae, but the old 'primary' holds and perpetuates the pattern.

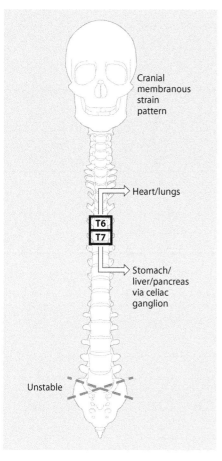

Cranial membranous strain pattern

Heart/lungs

T6
T7

Stomach/ liver/pancreas via celiac ganglion

Unstable

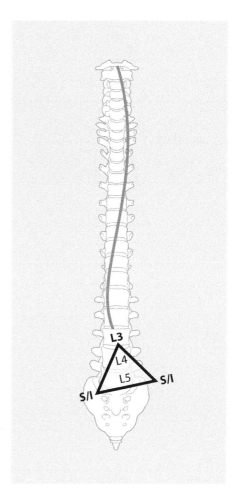

L3
L4
L5
S/I
S/I

Figure 8 notes

Here we see two principles expressed: the first is that chronic structural dysfunctions (e.g. intracranial birth patterns, traumatic or otherwise), can establish predisposing weaknesses extending throughout the body so that future somatic dysfunctions become more likely (a principle on which prophylaxis is based). Secondly, that segmental facilitation will often 'spill over' to involve 3-4 spinal segments through 'spread of excitation' such that too inflexible a view of the somatico-visceral distribution of effect is to be discouraged. These represent but two facets of a possibly more complex total lesion.

Figure 9 notes

The L3-sacro-iliac 'triangle' is itself a demonstration of functional reciprocity in which the mechanical functioning of L3, L4, L5 and the sacro-iliac joints are interdependent. Many different corrective approaches reflecting different diagnostic models can be effective in restoring normal function to this 'triangle', though each model places emphasis on different structural components within it.

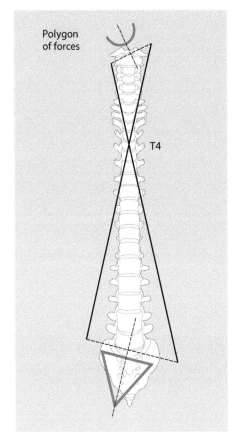

Polygon of forces

T4

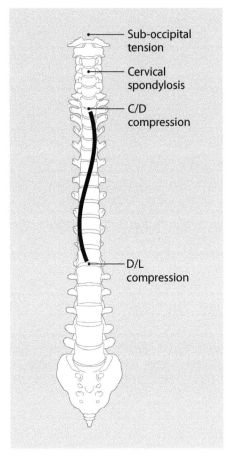

Sub-occipital tension

Cervical spondylosis

C/D compression

D/L compression

Figure 10 notes

The 'Polygon of Forces': According to the classical model of spinal mechanics, the anterior and posterior gravity lines relating to spinal function create a tensional network, crossing anteriorly to T4. This effectively creates two 'triangles'(or more accurately, pyramids) with their respective apices at this T4 level. (This can vary according to the antero-posterior balance of the individual spine and might, in severe kyphosis, for example, be two or three segments lower.) In practice, the T4 functionally co-ordinates and integrates upper and lower triangles and can often assume primacy to destabilize (or reflect) the cranio-cervical and lumbo-sacral complexes.

Figure 11 notes

A significant kyphoscoliosis can affect the intrathoracic and intra-abdominal viscera through altered cavity pressures and their effects on circulation and drainage. But it can also alter musculoskeletal functioning more widely, producing, for example, compression and hypomobility at cervico-dorsal and dorso-lumbar junctions, altered neck posture and mechanics, exacerbating a tendency to degenerative changes (cervical spondylosis) and cranio-cervical tension plus potential effects on the contents of the jugular foramina (vagus and spinal accessory nerves and jugular veins).

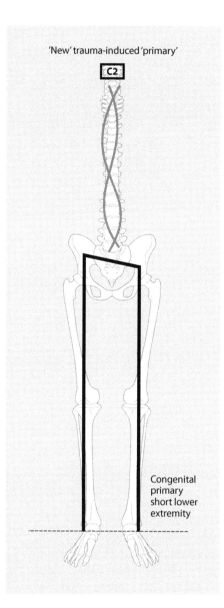

'New' trauma-induced 'primary'

C2

Congenital
primary
short lower
extremity

Figure 12 notes

Another example of 'two primaries': 1. The
primary short lower extremity, well-
compensated. 2. The more recent upper
cervical trauma-induced lesion with its
own 'layer' of compensatory changes.
These 'layers' naturally coalesce.

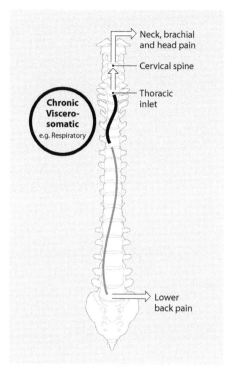

Neck, brachial
and head pain

Cervical spine

Thoracic
inlet

Chronic
Viscero-
somatic
e.g. Respiratory

Lower
back pain

Figure 13 notes

Complex interacting viscero-somatic and
somatico-somatic reflex cycles. Here, we
postulate a case of chronic respiratory illness
with raised facilitation of upper thoracic
spinal segments and disturbance of vertebral motion patterns as well as costo-verte-
bral, diaphragmatic, dorso-lumbar, scalene
and cervico-thoracic spinal functions.
Consequent effects of these 'secondaries'
may be reflected in head and neck pain, just
as the instability produced through the
spine as a whole can disturb lumbo-sacral
integrity with resultant back pain. The illusion of several different 'ailments' here can
be rationalised by this sustaining pattern
based in 'structure'. A holistic approach can
therefore work towards a resolution in all
respects as the various symptoms expressed
are interwoven in the structural patterning
as a whole.

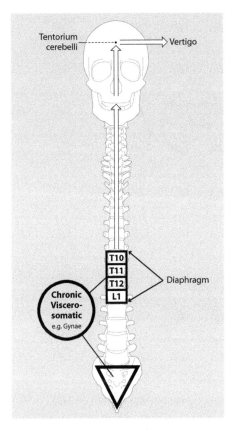

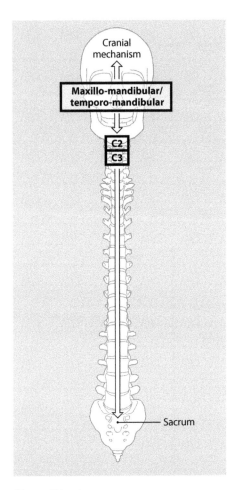

Figure 14 notes

The dynamic in this example demonstrates a similar principle to the last pattern although it is based on an altogether different clinical picture. A chronic gynaeco-logical problem, e.g. dysmenorrhea, uterine fibroids, endometriosis reflected in irritable viscero-somatic pathways centred on the sympathetic and parasympathetic supplies to the intrapelvic viscera. The pattern shows the secondary effects of the lower thoracic and sacral dysfunctions on the diaphragm and intracranial membranes (reciprocal tension) plus the hypothesised consequence of abnormal tentorial movement giving rise to vertigo. A general exacerbating malaise develops as these symptoms progressively erode constitutional health and resistance.

Figure 15 notes

The all-important dental component in which the maxillo-mandibular occlusion has potentially profound orthopaedic and osteopathic effects on the body as a whole via its influence on the functioning of the entire craniosacral mechanism. This occlusal phenomenon can be perceived osteopathically as another 'articulation' (with the property of circumduction). The neuromuscular correlates of this, along with the neuromuscular consequences of dental procedures themselves, can be highly significant in the formation of the 'total lesion'.

REFERENCES

Blechschmidt, E, 1978, *Biokinetics and Biodynamics of Human Differentiation*, Springfield.

Hall, TE, (1956), *Physiological Movement of the Spine*, Osteopathic Institute of Applied Technique.

Ho, M-W, 2008, *The Rainbow and the Worm*, World Scientific Publishing.

Ingber, D, 2008, Tensegrity and mechanotransduction, *Journal of Bodywork and Movement Therapies* 12:198–200.

Leach, B, 1975, *The Potter's Challenge*, Souvenir Press.

Levin, S, 1982, Continuous tension, discontinuous compression, a model for biomechanical support of the body, *Bulletin of Structural Integration* 8(2), 31–33, Rolf Institute.

Littlejohn, J M, 1956, *Development of the Spine*, Osteopathic Institute of Applied Technique.

Parsons, J & Marcer, N, 2006, *Osteopathy*, Churchill Livingstone.

Stapp, H, 1971, S-matrix interpretation of quantum theory, *Physical Review* D3, 1303–1320.

Wernham, S G J, 1956, *Mechanics of the Spine*, Osteopathic Institute of Applied Technique.

Chapter 5

From Mainstream to 'Cranial': continuum or quantum leap?

Here we look at a spectrum of osteopathic styles and the false distinctions made between them (as well as some of the real ones).

In about 1980, it was suggested that I teach an introductory course in 'cranial osteopathy' to our 3rd year students at the European School of Osteopathy (ESO). I was somewhat flattered as my 'cranial' experience was rather limited at that time. However, it had become so profoundly integrated into my thinking by then and it must have been thought that I had some facility with the approach, and so I was asked. My enthusiasm for the work was enormous but my compulsion was to introduce the students to the approach as a part of the overall osteopathic concept, not as a separate branch of our discipline.

This was so important to me that I justified my teaching it at all on the basis that I would teach an integrative approach, and that we were introducing the concept at undergraduate level. This was new in the UK at that time as previously 'cranial' work – or IVM (Involuntary Mechanism) studies as it is now more usually termed – was offered as a postgraduate option and was taken up by a distinct minority of the graduate profession. It was wonderfully championed by Colin Dove (former principal of the BSO) who imported much of the style and content of the Sutherland Cranial Teaching Foundation in the USA and taught courses annually in the UK from 1973/4.

What I was doing was controversial. It was felt, especially by those in the faculty who were unsympathetic and unskilled in IVM work, that students should study the 'mainstream' (whatever that was), and wander off into 'esoteric' realms after graduating if they so wished. One could of course sympathise with the view that the inclusion of IVM in the curriculum was loading the course with more challenges as well as asking the students to train themselves in a slightly different method of palpation along with the mindset that that required. I was of course 100 per cent in favour despite the challenges posed and still say to this day that students should explore the 'cranial' field even if they don't intend to use it later; it will enhance their palpation, their structural technique and allow them to explore the osteopathic concept in ever greater depth.

The point here is that, contrary to the assertions of some, so-called 'cranial' work and so-called 'mainstream' osteopathy are conceptual bedfellows even if they are procedurally different and sometimes call for different types of palpatory ability and intellectual approach. For even within the profession, prejudice abounds and is expressed on both sides of the (illusory) 'cranial' divide: the 'anti' crowd seeing 'cranial' as some kind of unfounded delusion; the 'cranial' lobby often seeing anything else as interventionist and depriving the body of its capacity for prioritised response patterns. These flawed positions create a totally artificial conceptual division and are based on superficial perspectives in both cases. So let's firstly look at what these approaches share and then we can move on to celebrate their differences.

Common Threads

Dr Still must have been aware that the principles he elaborated as the foundation for osteopathic thinking could well relate to the body as a totality, including the skull. He asked one of his gifted students, Charlotte Weaver, to research this in relation to the anatomy, embryology and neurology of the brain and cranial structures and this she did over many years, publishing her findings in the *Journal of the American Osteopathic Association* in 1936. Her researches centred very much on the notochord, pituitary gland and its anatomical home – the *sella turcica*. But the principle of structure/function reciprocity was to be extrapolated much more widely and the theory was elaborated significantly of course by Dr William Garner Sutherland who is considered to be the father of 'osteopathy in the cranial field'.

For many reasons, the 'cranial osteopathic' concept has been the source of tremendous debate and controversy both inside and outside the profession. Despite much of the almost poetic rhetoric that we find in much of the early writing on the subject, along with the over-emphasis on 'mechanical' analogy, many of the best informed and deepest thinkers in the profession have espoused the 'cranial' model and much of what has been elaborated in the field of 'energy medicine' research has fortified the model quite remarkably.

However, the subtle and, for some, elusive aspect of 'cranial' theory and practice has led detractors to consider it lacking in rationale and dependent instead on intuition and a 'spiritual' dimension. Whatever contribution these qualities might lend this field, its rational foundation is as strong as in any other osteopathic method.

There can be very little doubt that many of the pioneers of osteopathy, from Still himself, along with many of their followers, have been imbued with a sense of the numinous, many of their ideas being permeated by spiritual notions that have been reflected in their writing. Although this has largely been balanced by the spirit of analysis and rational enquiry, it has, over the years, caused those of a more pragmatic nature to denigrate the teachings of these fine minds, fostering a division in the profession and a reluctance to look deeper at the wisdom enfolded in such ideas. Whereas science, philosophy and the numinous were intertwined prior to the era of the Enlightenment, we have experienced a gradual de-coupling of these fields of human endeavour and enquiry and the dominance of rationality over the experiential and intuitive persist to this day.

SWEDENBORG

Emanuel Swedenborg (1688–1772) was a scientist, a philosopher, a theologian, an inventor, and a Christian mystic. He was said to have influenced many great thinkers including Blake, Goethe, Balzac, Jung, Kant, Strindberg, Yeats and many others. Much of his thinking on spiritual matters and the role of the spiritual dimension in the human realm have echoes in the later contributions of Still and Sutherland. But some of Swedenborg's ideas in relation to the body and the skull, brain and spine have remarkable resonances with the work of W.G. Sutherland, and it is widely believed that Swedenborg's ideas that were translated and elaborated by Rudolf Tafel (1831–1893) in *The Brain* (Swedenborg & Tafel, 1882) formed the basis of Sutherland's thinking in his formulation of the 'cranial' concept and what he termed the 'primary respiratory mechanism'.

Here are some of Swedenborg's ideas in this area that are fascinating to any student of osteopathy in the cranial field. From experiments performed on dogs, he remarked on the inherent motion characteristics of the brain and the rhythmic extrusion of cerebrospinal fluid from the brain. Anticipating what Sutherland would later refer to as 'the breath of life' and 'the fluid within the fluid', Swedenborg saw the location of the 'life force' to be in the fluid 'between the fibres', or what we would now see as the fluid matrix comprising the ground substance or extracellular matrix. He also believed that the brain was 'contractile' and, in its motion, was responsible for pumping this 'vital force'. Along with his theories on the dura and the cranial sutures that 'absorb' and restrain the effects of the brain's expansion, it is irresistible to consider the source of Sutherland's thinking in Swedenborg's writing that predated the publication of *The Cranial Bowl* by over 50 years (Sutherland, 1939).

The cranial concept on the osteopathic spectrum

Osteopathy's basic tenets regarding 'structure' and 'function' and their interdependency apply equally to the cranium (and the 'craniosacral' mechanism) as well as to the rest of the musculoskeletal system. Mechanisms of dysfunction are 'read' in both instances through assessment of motion and 'vitality'; in other words, the quality, direction and range of movement in a structure are parameters that are assessed both for themselves AND in relation to other structures with which they are in relationship.

However, the quality of motion in the skull and its associated tissues and structures is clearly different from the patterns of *gross* movement usually assessed in other parts of the body (both musculoskeletal and otherwise). But here, two points should be made: the first is that 'cranial' motion is a palpable quality extending throughout *all* body structures if one chooses to look for it. And secondly, the abnormalities of motion on both of these 'osteopathic' dimensions are potentially equally related to altered physiological function and therefore qualify as 'osteopathic' in the same degree. In reality, of course, they are part of a seamless unity.

These physiological effects relate to fluid dynamics and neural function, again whether looking at the 'cranial' or 'non-cranial' sphere. Some of these fluid dynamics relate to 'fluid fluctuation', a phenomenon that is palpable in both spheres, whether we are speaking of cerebrospinal fluid fluctuation in the cranio-spinal domain or of Still's 'withering fields' and their dependency upon the efficient 'irrigation' and drainage of tissues via the fascia and interstitial fluid throughout the entire body.

To reiterate, the subtle manifestations of motility, the rhythmic ebb and flow of tissue vitality, are palpable anywhere in the body but, by and large, the discipline of 'structural' osteopathy prioritises larger amplitude movements and consequently a different mental and palpatory orientation such that 'cranial' motion and all that that connotes is often rejected or ignored by some exponents of that particular osteopathic 'style'. The fact remains that the 'cranial' concept is in truth not defined by its regional, anatomical significance, but by its notion of integrated motility as a whole body phenomenon based on the characteristics of the connective tissue matrix and its bioelectric properties.

DIFFERENCES

Without doubt, the palpatory and manual methods employed in cranial work are somewhat different from the classical or 'structural' approach. One might say that they are a different way of 'listening'. Furthermore, this is not just a matter of subtlety; it is not impossible to find heavy-handed and unsubtle cranial practitioners and superbly skilled and subtle 'structuralists'; so no superiority in terms of skills is implied in either direction.

But here it gets interesting. Structural treatment usually involves a range of physical skills directed at skeletal and soft tissue, whether muscle, ligament, tendon or fascia. These techniques might involve pressure (light or otherwise), rhythmic articulatory movements applied to joints or joint manipulation, usually of high velocity and low amplitude producing the stereotypical cavitation 'pop' so loved or despised by patients, or various positioning techniques with or without active muscle involvement.

Cranial technique on the other hand is very different, both to observe and to experience, for it would seem, on the surface, to involve little more than touch or the 'laying on of hands'. The extent to which this 'touch' is informed is hard to overestimate, for it is based on a remarkably sensitive connection with a highly assimilated knowledge of anatomy as well as a grasp of the significance physiologically and otherwise of changes in function. When these skills are first acquired, the changes in function are categorised within a framework known as the 'five phenomena' of Sutherland. Like so much in osteopathic teaching, this provides a conceptual approach to the understanding or processing of our palpatory findings. The connection is made with structure through a form of touch that can 'travel' as the practitioner dictates through the projection of his or her mental connection with the patient's 'material' (their functioning anatomy and its significance in more general terms). The effects of this contact are extraordinary as the practitioner establishes a virtually 'pivotal' contact with particular structures as choices are strategically made in response to the diagnosed pattern, both in structural and clinical terms. Many have felt that this 'connection' is only possible through some kind of awareness of a 'field', a field reflecting bioelectric energy, expressing in an oscillatory or rhythmic manner. (This oscillatory field and our interaction with it is where quantum theory becomes relevant). Meanwhile, the matter of rhythm or rhythmicity is a phenomenon that has somewhat different resonances when comparing 'structural' with cranial osteopathy.

Rhythm

In structural work, the rhythm is imposed through skilful articulation, and good rhythm is spoken of as evidenced by good trophicity or healthy trophic function in tissues. In cranial work, we both listen to and promote or release patterned rhythmic motility in bone, membrane and even in fluid fluctuation. The importance of rhythmic oscillation in living tissue is unquestionable and such oscillations have been discussed in Chapter 2 with, for example, the contribution of Herbert Fröhlich. The significance of rhythm in the cranial concept is, of course, mostly articulated in discussion of the 'cranial rhythm', the cranial rhythmic impulse or the concept of 'primary respiration'. This concept on its own has created enough controversy, particularly as regards the matter of the origin of this motion (again, recall Chapter 2). Meanwhile, it is worth recounting Sutherland's basic tenets, or 'the five phenomena' as they are termed, which became the template with which to 'read' the patient in the cranial osteopathic model. These are, of course, well-known to aficionados, but help round out the picture for everyone else. Once more, these need to be seen as signposts or working tools to be fashioned into a model. In other words, they need to be interpreted. I'll quote them as they are originally posed, but then I'd like to quote Paul Lee's reinterpretation which modulates them beautifully. They are:

- Inherent motility of the central nervous system
- Fluctuation of cerebrospinal fluid
- Mobility of the intracranial and intraspinal dural membranes
- Mobility of the cranial bones
- Mobility of the sacrum between the ilia

Lee then distils these 'five phenomena' into the following two-part summary of the 'cranial' concept:

1. A palpable oscillation of the central nervous system occurs with the fluctuation of electrolytes and water between the intracellular and extracellular compartments.
2. Accommodation for this primary initiative occurs with passive motion of the cranial bones, the sacrum, and the reciprocating dural membranes, the latter serving to integrate all motions of the bones surrounding the CNS.

Then, entirely appropriately, Lee expands the concept to include the totality of body function as follows:

1. The movement of water and electrolytes creates alternating sol and gel phases of the extracellular matrix that coincide with contraction and swelling phases, respectively, of the parenchymal cells, and delivers nutrients and removes waste products appropriately as the basis for metabolism.
2. The connective tissues display the characteristics of piezoelectricity and tensegrity as a means by which they biomechanically accommodate and participate in oscillating fluid metabolism (Lee, 2005).

Here, the sense of an integrated patterned oscillation throughout the body and manifesting in all tissues, fluids and structures (though varying qualitatively depending on where we 'look'), seems much more real than the more linear, over-mechanical model in which one type of movement is said to 'drive' another. Fundamentally however, Sutherland emphasised the rhythmic 'tidal motion' of the extracellular and cerebrospinal fluids as the vehicle for the 'potency' or vitality that generates healthy physiology. (Such references on the part of both Still and Sutherland almost intimate the expression or even the seat of 'consciousness' itself!) Though exponents highlight various 'tides' manifesting throughout the body (just as there are many oscillatory rates in different tissues, organs etc.), the tide that most practitioners work with in the cranial field is an 8–12 per minute cycle, though the rate – along with that of the 'long tide' – is not hugely significant; its quality, distribution and expression are.

But as with everything in osteopathy, the 'cranial' concept is also subject to different interpretations or different 'hues'. Some work very comfortably with a 'mechanical' model that aligns itself more closely with Sutherland's teaching. Others espouse the 'biodynamic' concept so beautifully developed by James Jealous based on his research into the metabolic fields expressed by the embryo and supported by the work of Erich Blechschmidt MD (1978). In this way, Jealous links the 'generative' forces expressed in the embryo during development with the rhythmically expressed regenerative forces in any organism's pattern of healing and repair; this is of course the potential that we attempt to access and facilitate in treatment, and it parallels what Still meant when he said that the task of the doctor is 'to find health' ('anyone can find disease').

A false lead

As I mentioned at the outset, osteopathy is riddled with misconceptions, both inside and outside the profession. As regards the 'cranial' concept, one of the many false premises is the oversimplification that the cranial model is *dependent* on the existence of cranial bone motion, i.e. motion between the bones at their sutures. The 'cranial debate' raged for years over this vital point as to whether the anatomists were right in their assertion that the cranial bones fused through the process of ossification and was more or less complete by the age of 18–25 years, allowing for no motion whatsoever and thus invalidating the concept.

In the late 1970s, Dr John Upledger carried out research with Dr. Ernest Retzlaff on the histology of the cranial sutures (Retzlaff & Mitchell, 1987) and revealed through complex staining techniques that the suture architecture was quite clearly designed to permit and sustain an element of motion throughout life, even though that movement was of course very slight. There was also much mention of the Italian schools of anatomy that had historically taught an alternative view that sutural motion was not completely obliterated by the process of maturation. What's more, it appeared that the sutural physiology itself was connected reflexly with the brain and the intracranial dura such that the 'structure/function' exchange was as likely to operate here as anywhere else in the body.

Now as significant as this was, it side-stepped the issue of inherent, universal oscillatory or rhythmic motion – what Sutherland called 'primary respiration' – in all living tissue; and as all 'cranial' practitioners know, *intraosseous* motion, or the lack of it, is every bit as significant as *interosseous* motion which, in turn, is as important as all the various fluctuant waves of motion throughout all Sutherland's 'five phenomena' as well as every tissue and cell in the body. This ubiquitous wave of fluctuation manifesting variously, depending on which structures or tissues are under scrutiny, AND the extent to which these motions are integrated, or 'orchestrated', combine to produce the expression of 'primary respiration' that reflect the health and vitality of the organism. And it is potentially detectable anywhere: in bone, in muscle, ligament, membrane, cartilage . . . anywhere.

As we saw in Chapter 2 on mobility, different tissues express motion in different ways as they transmute energy differently depending on morphology, genetic structure and function. The quality of sutural motion is different from that of intraosseous motion, and so the type of 'strain pattern' that occurs will reflect this, just as it will reflect the embryological development of the structure concerned coupled, of course, with the effects of the patient's particular historical details.

Certain areas in the spine and cranium alike are particularly susceptible to strain or injury. As Tom Dummer (1995) expressed most emphatically, it is both the *morphology* as well as the *location* of the upper cervical and lumbosacral complexes that make them more prone to the *positional,* traumatically-induced lesion, taking them beyond restriction of mobility to a potential spatial mal-relationship; relatively unusual in the realm of spinal lesions generally, but common in relation to trauma. This is often crucial in the osteopathic clinical situation in which the 'positional adjustment' may be therapeutically paramount.

Similarly, in the cranium, there are areas of particular vulnerability too, though strain patterns in the mechanism can be found almost anywhere in the body. However, birth injuries and obstetric complications, e.g. difficult or protracted labour, abnormal presentations, forceps or ventouse deliveries and birth by Caesarian section, as well as intrauterine compressions prior to birth, all have attendant risks in the creation of compressions and vectors that distort the normal pattern and distribution of 'cranial' motion. Furthermore, certain areas are, by virtue of position and morphology, prone to complex strain patterns that require special attention as they form special pivotal or 'speed-reducing' roles in the interlocking anatomical parts of the cranial mechanism (e.g. the spheno-squamous pivot and the zygomatico-temporal suture).

The concept of 'primary respiration' transcends the debate as to whether or not the skull bones move – of course they do – but the quality of the movement between them is different from the quality of the movement *within* them. But those who take issue with the matter of sutural mobility might struggle even more with the whole concept of 'primary respiration'. Meanwhile, motion in living organisms manifests in many ways. The subtle oscillations that reflect the quality of 'aliveness' are as significant as the movement of blood through our arteries, even where these movements are only palpable through a specialised perceptual process. The question then arises as to whether these movements are mechanical or are the expression of oscillating 'fields', and what exactly it is that we palpate therefore (see Chapter 7).

FIELDS

We refer briefly to 'field theory' in Chapter 7, from the early cultural traditions to the more contemporary theories of Burr, Sheldrake and Rein, and when we yoke these notions to what we know about the connective tissue matrix, its bioelectric properties and its influence on cell function via the cytoskeletal network, a picture begins to emerge that illuminates both the cranial and wider osteopathic concept.

Indeed, our understanding of the structure and function of living tissues has altered radically through the contributions of contemporary biologists and physicists who have examined the function of tissue in the light of quantum theory and the crystalline qualities of the collagen and water molecules that comprise connective tissue (Szent-Györgyi , 1957). Here, the parallels between the semiconductor 'switching' properties of cell membranes and those of the microchip are interesting to ponder as we incorporate the notion of the membrane informationally and metabolically mediating the extracellular 'environment' and the cell interior. In this way, the influence of the extracellular matrix, both physiologically and bioelectrically, on cell function, including protein patterning or *conformation* and gene expression, is enormously significant (Lipton 2005, Ingber 1997, 2008). This challenge to the notion of 'gene supremacy' recalls the much maligned theory of Jean-Baptiste Lamarck who not only held that genetic expression could be modulated by adaptive behaviour, but also that the acquired pattern of gene expression could be passed on to the inheriting progeny. More recently, Ingber's writing on tensegrity and mechanotransduction challenges the momentum of gene-based theory in disease causation to highlight the importance of biomechanical forces to the biological control of molecules and cells (Ingber, 2008).

FASCIA

Though Still had emphasised the significance of fascia in a remarkably insightful view of physiological function and the contribution that the body structure makes to it, it has been in the theoretical sphere of IVM that fascia and the connective tissue matrix of which it is part have really proclaimed a dominant role. This is partly based on the importance of fascial continuity and its significance to the concept of 'reciprocal tension', and partly based on the bioelectric properties of collagen and water within connective tissue, and their relevance to the 'cranial' model. Indeed, their significance is considerable and their influence ubiquitous, as Jane Stark expresses in her excellent articles on fascia in *Osteopathy Today* (Feb 2011):

> *'Fascia responds to a whole array of internal and external*
> *environmental stimuli, including pressure gradients, tension fields,*
> *nutrient (inorganic and organic) availability (in the liquid matrix)*

and assimilation, vascularisation, as well as neural stimulation or lack thereof. It reacts to the addition and withdrawal of mechanical, chemical and thermal, pharmacological, electromagnetic, and even emotional stimuli. Finally, if water is absent, the only sure reaction is cellular death; none of fascia's purposeful reactions can take place, including the production and arrangement of its fibres.'

Now clearly, the importance of connective tissue and all its properties are not exclusive to the cranial approach; Still's emphasis on fascia obviously predated Sutherland's pioneering work in the cranial field. But in 'mainstream' osteopathy, the fascia has been rather neglected although none of its exponents would eliminate the fascia from the sphere of influence of the musculoskeletal system *per se* and their therapeutic approach to it. Indeed, it is my view that the connective tissue matrix is common to all strands of the osteopathic theory and the 'dialogue' with 'function', no matter which osteopathic model is adopted.

THE MATRIX

The conventional view of connective tissue, including fascia, is of some kind of ubiquitous 'packing material' both separating and lending support to other structures, including the viscera. Occasionally it has been conceded that it might also have some contractile function independent of muscle but this has not generally been widely asserted.

The 'living' quality and influence of the connective tissue 'system' or matrix has been beautifully articulated by James Oschman (2000). Here, Oschman pays tribute to the remarkable work of anatomist Alfred Pischinger (1899–1982) on the extracellular matrix and its role in biological regulation. His work almost echoes Still and his emphasis on 'fascia' as the anatomical 'repository' for the regulation of health, compromises of which are the precursor to dysfunction and disease. With Pischinger's *The Extracellular Matrix and Ground Regulation* (2007), we not only have a superb new edition of his work, clearly showing the significance of this concept to many holistic systems of practice, but also a wonderful contribution to our osteopathic model that underpins the spectrum of osteopathic thought, once again blurring the false distinctions so often drawn between the various orientations and interpretations.

As we've seen in Chapter 1, there are some ideas that are so central to osteopathic practice, it is interesting that they have until recently only been hinted at, without much validation. So, let us look a little deeper at the fascinating world of the connective tissue and the 'living' matrix along with the extracellular space, what it comprises and the relevance to us here. It is worth mentioning at this point that Oschman, alluding to the functional interconnection with the connective tissue interior of the cell and the cytoskeleton, coins the term 'living matrix' to incorporate the whole. Furthermore, Pischinger himself was asserting the importance of the connective tissue when he stated:

> 'The concept of a cell is, strictly speaking, only a morphological abstraction. Seen from a purely biological viewpoint, a cell cannot be considered by itself without taking its environment into account'
>
> (Pischinger, 2007)

It is also worth remembering that it is the physiology of the extracellular space that links the body's nerves and capillaries with the cells themselves which they do not access directly.

Connective tissue qualities

Connective tissue arises or is formed from embryonic mesoderm and is characterised by a highly vascularised matrix including collagen, elastic and reticular fibres, adipose tissue, cartilage and bone. And as Oschman's survey of it recalls (2000):

- The connective tissue fabric or matrix unifies the body and all its systems as it is a mechanical continuum extending throughout the entire body and into the innermost parts of each cell via *integrins* and other transmembrane linking molecules.
- It determines the shape of the organism as well as the detailed architecture of its parts.
- All movement, whether of the whole body or of its smallest parts, is created by tensions carried through the matrix.
- Each tension, each compression, each movement causes the crystalline lattice of the connective tissues to generate bioelectronic signals that are precisely characteristic of those tensions, compressions and movements.
- The connective tissue fabric is a semiconducting communication network that can carry bioelectronic signals between every part of the body and every other part.

Clearly, these properties are far richer, far more complex than the simple 'packing material' image more generally taught, and they cast Still's insights concerning 'structure/function' connections in a most remarkable light with their properties of semi-conduction, piezoelectricity, crystallinity, coherency, hydration, continuity, tensegrity and information storage, processing and transfer.

Looking a little closer, the micro-architecture of the extracellular space contains elements of connective tissue including fascia and the extracellular matrix, often referred to as the 'ground substance', extracellular fluid, and a network of capillaries, lymphatics and nerve endings, all impacting cell function.

The emphasis in medicine and physiology on mechanisms based in and on the surface of the cell has largely ignored the vital role of the extracellular space on the health and survival of the cells themselves. And, as Paul Lee reminds us, this extracellular space functions as a filter, a primitive nervous system, a whole body registry, an immune system, a storage compartment, a system of integrating 'structure', a unifying system, a detoxifying system and a medium for regulating cell function by hormones, polypeptides, inflammatory intermediates etc.

The extracellular matrix itself with its complex meshwork of structural glycoproteins (including collagen, elastin and fibronectin) constitutes a molecular sieve through which all the processes of cellular metabolism percolate (Lee, 2005).

The function of this matrix, as part of the complex electrically-charged machinery of the body framework, is what links 'structure' and 'function' together in a physiological union.

So the mechanical aspects of this unifying function are paralleled by the extraordinarily vital role that the connective tissue system plays in whole-body operations. And the bioelectrical information and signalling that this involves is as important to the functional integration of the body as it is to health and survival. As already stated, the electromagnetic charge patterns that are exchanged between the connective tissue matrix and the cell influence the conformation of intracellular proteins, extending to the nucleus and the DNA, challenging the received dogma of the primacy of the gene in cellular function (Lipton, 2005).

Recapping: quantum theory in relation to osteopathic holism

Now, returning to the significance of quantum theory for our osteopathic discipline: firstly, it elaborates the concept of interconnectedness – one of the planks of holism – in a remarkable way through the greater understanding of these semiconductor and piezoelectric properties of connective tissue, collagen and water. This expanded concept is based on the rapid information (photonic) transfer bioelectrically or bioenergetically through the body to produce functional integration; integration that is functionally intertwined with the tension/ compression elements in the tissues that make up the body framework – its 'tensegrous' property.

Secondly, this tensegrous patterning of the body structure generates bioelectrical signalling that communicates via the cell membrane and its semiconductor transmembrane proteins or integrins with the cytoskeletal structures and the cell nucleus. This not only impacts on intracellular physiology and metabolism but potentially, as suggested, modulates gene expression.

Thirdly, it underpins the holistic concept by which efficient physiological function – health – is seen as the product of *quantum coherence*, a feature that expresses itself through functional anatomy and physiology to influence connective tissue function and therefore cell biology. Such coherence, or lack of it, is reflected or interpreted through numerous schemata or models to be 'read' according to the protocols of different clinical disciplines *in their own terms*, osteopathy being just one such.

COHERENCE AND ENTRAINMENT

This coherence can be 'entrained' with the coherence generated in and by the practitioner whose knowledge and intention can be focussed in a method that 'engages' the patient's system; *practitioner coherence entrains patient coherence*. (I believe that there is an interesting parallel here with the concept and inculcation of *direction* in the Alexander Technique).

The concept of *entrainment* has many applications in physics and biology, but it is perhaps useful here to insert a brief description:

> *Most, if not all, biological and behavioural processes are rhythmic and cyclical in nature* (Oatley & Goodwin, 1971). *Entrainment refers to the process whereby an endogenous biological or behavioural rhythm is modified in its phase and periodicity by powerful exogenous influences*
> . . . (Ancona & Chong, 1992).

The coherent patterning is evaluated in our approach via the function of the anatomy and the 'structure/function bonds' already mentioned, mediated by the connective tissue matrix and its tensegrous operation, with its influence on the physiology of the extracellular spaces, cell membranes and cytoskeleton. This couples with the cranio-spinal system, and its relationship with the circulatory and neuro-endocrine systems. And this expression is largely 'read' in osteopathic practice through patterns of motion, motility and rhythmicity, as we consistently assert, however gross or subtle these patterns may be. The range of motion in both the axial and appendicular skeletal mechanisms is at the conspicuous end of the spectrum, whereas the qualities of motion expressed in subtler ways are represented in an extraordinary range of palpatory experiences in which the 'energy' expressed in tissues may feel 'intensified', 'depleted', 'irritable', poorly connected or integrated, in other words, 'alienated', 'scattered' and unfocussed, and even powerfully expressive of emotion: sadness, despair, fear, shock, etc. etc. (Pert, 1997).

It is worth stating that this 'coherence' factor is unconscious in the patient, whereas in the practitioner it is engendered as a product of technique. This technique is a mysterious blending of certain key elements: the practitioner's knowledge of 'normal' function as expressed through motion/motility patterns coupled with osteopathic principles (structure/function and mechanical inter-relationships), AND the ability to engage the body through a condition of complete balanced 'stillness'.

The practitioner creates an 'emptying', a state of physical and mental poise and stillness through which the connection is made, whilst at the same time carrying a blueprint for correction, a template with which the targeted tissues are able to 'entrain'. The beauty of the concept of the 'focus' or 'primary lesion' at the heart of the presenting pattern – 'the eye of the storm' – is that the entrainment of the part provides the potential for entrainment of the 'whole'.

The specific adjustment meanwhile contains similar ingredients but includes the projection of a physical corrective force or movement even though it is applied with a mindset that holds the total lesion in its sights up to the moment of correction; the therapeutic 'force' is *projected* rather than placed.

Voluntary or involuntary?

One conceptual argument that sometimes threatens to divide the 'cranial' fraternity from the rest revolves around the issue of the 'involuntary' nature of the Involuntary Mechanism, this relating ostensibly to its motility charac-teristics in contrast to those of the musculoskeletal system. Meanwhile several 'cranial' practitioners espouse the former concept with the implied propensity of the body to prioritise its own pattern of movement responses and sequences of correction. As attractive as this notion is, it can sometimes connote negli-gible input from the practitioner and an almost autonomous response on the part of the patient's 'mechanism'.

I would, however, point out that even in the realm of the apparently minimal intervention that 'cranial' work is, it is not a passive or purely 'listening' process; it is participatory; there are vital choices being made at every juncture by the practitioner which constantly alter the nature of the input and the calls on the body's responses. I expand on this in Chapter 7, 'The Intelligent Fulcrum'. In addition we must always remember the intertwining of the Involuntary Mechanism with the musculoskeletal and every other body system. As with everything else in osteopathy, we are looking at a continuum, a unit of func-tion through which work directed at one dimension is available to all others when properly applied. Furthermore, the body's prioritised responses are also elicited by 'structural' approaches to treatment.

CONCLUSION

As we've basked in a mechanistic age from the Enlightenment, through indus-trialisation and onwards into the twentieth and twenty-first centuries, the traditional and even archaic idea of 'energy' in medicine has been shunned.

And this has happened despite both Einstein and quantum theory leaving a continuum in therapeutics that is polarised between the apparent conceptual opposites of 'mechanism' and 'vitalism', the latter most commonly associated with the 'alternative' field.

Even within osteopathy, practice and theoretical orientation could be said to be split this way, with the 'mechanists' espousing formulaic 'evidence-based' practice, their 'vitalist' colleagues cast in the mould of quaint but 'outmoded eccentrics' from past centuries who might include Mesmer, Burr and others. Many will recognise the value of integrating these two apparently divergent approaches. Meanwhile, it is interesting to see how this 'electronic' age of nanotechnology and quantum theory on which it has depended – the age of the 'invisible' and of probability rather than certainty – has penetrated our world, revolutionised our technology and validated the 'energetic' principle in medicine. This principle is in fact as relevant to so-called 'classical' osteopathy as it is to 'cranial', but it is the cranial field that has 'commissioned' it, as it has recalled much of what Still was intimating decades earlier. What's more, it has been more difficult within the 'cranial' approach to continue to impute purely mechanical processes (though, in reality, these are inadequate in relation to the more 'mainstream' osteopathic field too).

The beauty of the cranial concept is that it yokes together Still's original tenets, the power of the potency in the fluctuation and oscillation inherent in Sutherland's concept, the quantum coherence as described by Szent-Györgyi and Mae-Wan Ho and others, and the unifying principle of 'structure' – all of it, in essence, underscoring osteopathic practice from the most subtle to the most 'mechanical', while embracing the 'intentional' participatory quality inherent in manual skill.

We as osteopaths touch the body to try to comprehend it in terms based on all the foregoing. For all our knowledge and understanding, it sometimes feels as if its unimaginable and holistic complexity threatens to elude us as we use palpatory techniques to get closer to this complex 'reality'. For that reason, there are many in the profession who feel safer with the mechanical paradigm that provides a more accessible shorthand, a method though that, for all its sense of greater certainty, may in fact yield something more approximate. How strange then that when we cast off and 'set sail' on the extraordinary exploration of the IVM, some of us feel a little closer to something more 'real'.

Whichever 'reality' is preferred, both are, of course, always present. If we favour the Newtonian variety, well, it holds perfectly well for comparatively large objects and movements with their large mass and small wave function; things that are conspicuous in our material world. But even here, the quantum dynamic resides; the wave awaiting 'collapse' by the conscious mind of the observer when the process of de-contextualising, entrainment, coherence and re-contextualising create the opportunity for therapeutic work at its most extraordinary. Above all, it allows for – even demands – the coalition of matter, motion and 'mind', at once so reminiscent of Still and so bang up-to-date.

Ultimately, the more we ponder the osteopathic 'idea' and its various modes of practice, the more we see that there *is* no quantum leap; where quantum principles apply to the function of living tissues and organisms, they are naturally at work whichever method you espouse and whether the practitioner is aware of them or not. Whereas the immediate objectives of treatment may appear to vary depending on one's approach, the interconnected nature of the body's 'layers' ensure that the ultimate objectives of these varied 'styles' converge, even though certain situations might call for a specific approach at times.

It is somewhat curious that many, from medical insurance companies to the general public, take issue with 'cranial' as if it's some kind of arcane belief system, for in reality, these same people are almost certainly unaware of the *modus operandi* of 'mainstream' osteopathy, as well as most other medical methods in the conventional and alternative arenas for that matter. But then the intolerance of many things in our culture is based on the illusions that reflect a 'selective acceptance'; often an illusion based either on a poor conception of how things really work or a belief in them based on custom or conventional opinion, too established to be questioned!

Genuine osteopathy is truly a seamless whole, and the apparent schism between methods can be exhilaratingly explored so that its wholeness can begin radiantly to come into view.

REFERENCES

Ancona, D & Chong, C L, 1992, *Cycles and synergy in organisational behaviour.* In: Colquhoun W P (ed) *Biological Rhythms & Human Performance*, Academic.

Blechschmidt, E, 1978, *Biokinetics and Biodynamics of Human Differentiation*, Springfield.

Dummer, T G, 1995, *Specific Adjusting Technique*, Jotom.

Ingber, D, 1997, Tensegrity: the architectural basis of cellular mechanotransduction, *Annual Review of Physiology* 59:575–599.

Ingber, D, 2008, Tensegrity and mechanotransduction, *Journal of Bodywork and Movement Therapies* 12:198–200.

Lee, R. Paul, 2005, *Interface: Mechanisms of Spirit in Osteopathy*, Stillness Press.

Lipton, B, 2005, *The Biology of Belief*, Hay House.

Oatley, K & Goodwin, B, 1971, Explanation and Investigation of biological rhythms. In: W P Colquhoun (ed) *Biological Rhythms & Human Performance*, Academic.

Oschman, J, 2000, *Energy Medicine*, Churchill Livingstone.

Pert, C, 1997, *The Molecules of Emotion*, Simon & Schuster.

Pischinger, A, 2007,*The Extracellular Matrix and Ground Regulation*, North Atlantic Books.

Retzlaff, E & Mitchell, F, 1987,*The Cranium and its Sutures*, Springer-Verlag.

Stark, J, *Popular ruts: fascia revisited*, Osteopathy Today, Feb 2011, 12–13.

Sutherland, W G, 1939, *The Cranial Bowl*, Free Press Company.

Swedenborg, E & Tafel, L, 1882, *The Brain considered anatomically, physiologically and philosophically*, James Spiers.

Szent-Györgyi, A, 1957, *Bioenergetics*, Academic Press.

Weaver, C, 1936, The Cranial Vertebrae, *Journal of the American)steopathic Association*, 37 (3), 328–336.

Part 2

The Art of It

Chapter 6
Subjectivity and the 'dance'

Reality is in the observations, not in the electron.

Heisenberg: *Physics and Philosophy* (1958)

Let's say that the world is in essence neutral – flat, empty, bereft of meaning and significance. It's us, our imaginations, that make it vivid, fill it with colour, feeling, purpose and emotion. Once we understand this we can shape our world in any way we want. In theory.

William Boyd: *Waiting for Sunrise* (2012),
after Henri Bergson's *La Fonction Fabulatrice.*

The many concepts that distinguish osteopathy from other disciplines give us 'method', a virtual way-in to diagnosis and the treatment that follows. However, our conceptual framework is simply that: a scaffold on to which many other cues and clues have to be hung in order to see the patient more completely.

These details are what I sometimes mean as 'context'; the complexity that allows for the individuated expression of any given symptom or syndrome.

It is a cliché we should never tire of affirming: that the mechanism by which any given condition is expressed can vary from patient to patient. Likewise, a particular structural configuration may express itself in different symptoms in different patients. So, for example, the same structural dysfunction in the cranio-cervical complex might relate to headache in one patient, nausea and vertigo in another, excessive fatigue and 'vagotonia' in another. And as if that were not enough, because of the expression of reciprocity of function throughout the entire structural system, it might produce secondary effects that create their own reflex related sequelae. Compensatory structural changes sit at the heart of their own physiologically related consequences to form a complex meshwork of illness, sometimes with so many facets, that the illusion of multiple diseases or syndromes would appear to present (see Figs. 13 and 14 in Chapter 4).

Some might consider that this inconsistency invalidates the whole concept. Far from it. It underscores the uniqueness of the individual such that any given syndrome may well have a highly individuated mechanism of production and expression; the commonalities – i.e. where diseases share common features across a range of patients – are merely the beginning. This is one key point of distinction between holistic methods and some conventional allopathic perspectives.

Furthermore, it is largely through an appraisal of and response to the many contextual details in the patient's history and make-up that we come to prioritise the observed and palpated material in the session and devise a treatment plan or strategy that 'fits' the individual patient.

However, this is but one aspect of the unique 'dance' that is the patient/ practitioner exchange. And as in many dances, the partners have different interlocking roles. These roles are polarised: patient and practitioner are not equals in this gigue. The situation does, of course, demand a certain mutuality in terms of respect and in the sharing of certain common goals (patient benefit for example), but in other respects, the situation is one in which the roles are clearly different. The patient attends with his/her brief: a request for help; certain expectations based on experience or a lack of it; prejudices, misconceptions or sometimes unrealistically high hopes, and a variety of mindsets.

And what of the practitioner?

Practitioners too are individuals, unique, sometimes flawed and with 'baggage'. Hopefully our training and experience filter out the unhelpful bits to leave us with a set of skills and perspectives that are malleable to the individual patient and the unique circumstance of the consultation. Those skills have been honed to create abilities that become personalised, so that the practitioner gravitates towards a diagnostic perspective, method and technique (based on aptitude as well as orientation). Ideally we also learn to work from a place of 'neutrality' and non-judgement.

In the making of the practitioner, compassion and empathy sit alongside the ability to juxtapose an assimilation of the patient's wholeness with something of one's own humanity. It is a process of identification with a deeper struggle, a 'brokenness' that expresses itself through 'structure', and we ask how and why should these symptoms come to be expressed? What do they reflect? What kind of opportunity do they provide if sympathetically and holistically diagnosed and treated? How should we best engage them?

The individual practitioner's responses to any clinical presentation may be as individuated as the patient's expression of their problem. And here lies one of the vital ingredients of 'the dance': the subjectivity that is fundamental to any creative skill; an ingredient of great value. It is one's chosen method, its conceptual model and its 'rules' that govern what is 'seen' and prioritised in diagnosis. Every therapeutic system produces its own diagnostic template with a treatment strategy that is tailored from it, and ten different methods will 'reveal' ten different patterns. Yet any given patient's body 'contains' or expresses them all; all are true. It is our own particular orientation that yokes the clinical fact and detail to a subjectively driven approach. And within osteopathy itself, several 'orientations' exist; examples of these are misleadingly called 'techniques' as in 'structural technique', 'functional technique', 'specific adjusting technique' and 'cranial or craniosacral technique' which, as treatment approaches, comprise their own diagnostic systems as well as their own therapeutic procedures.

This will appear contrary to so much in medical (and some 'osteopathic') thinking as we contradict the trend to exclude, 'factor out', control for the subjective as though it were an irrelevance or a hindrance? Let's look further at this.

ALLOWING THE SUBJECTIVE IN

The contribution of subjectively-based inspiration to the advancement of scientific progress is well-established. In *The Logic of Scientific Discovery* Karl Popper (1934) placed the constructive creative guess of the scientist in its rightful role. Whilst maintaining the notion of science's rationality, its rigour and neutrality, he argued 'that it did not, as commonly thought, proceed by the systematic and cumulative collection of empirically verified facts. It moved forward when scientists came up with bold, imaginative guesses that could never be perfectly verified and were no more reliable than any other "belief" . . .' (Armstrong, 2009). So the relationship of subjectively based insights to notions of reality is compelling.

Reality

The insights given to us as quantum theory has gained momentum are an echo of the perennial philosophical preoccupation with the nature of *reality*. The assertion that there is no objective reality is counter-intuitive, for even if we accept quite rightly that all things have meaning in terms of the way they are perceived and cognitively processed, we still like to believe that there is an objective reality underneath.

The philosopher Immanuel Kant (1724–1804) was always aware of the limitations of Newton's mathematical 'logic', and he divided knowledge into three: appearance, reality and theory, neatly summarised by Nick Herbert in his book *Quantum Reality* (1985):

> *Appearance is the content of our direct sensory experience of natural phenomena. Reality (Kant called it the 'thing-in-itself') is what lies behind all phenomena. Theory consists of human concepts that attempt to mirror both appearance and reality . . . Kant believed that the world's appearances were deeply conditioned by human sensory and intellectual apparatus . . . Scientific facts – the appearances themselves – are as much a product of the observer's human nature as they are of an underlying reality. We see the world through particularly human goggles.*

Nowadays, many who speak about such things will impute the role of quantum theory in our concept of 'reality', and they will be used to the refrain: 'Ah, but quantum theory is only applicable to the sub-atomic, to the very small; everything else is subject to the laws of classical Newtonian physics'. Well, one might reply firstly that the 'very large' is inevitably and incontrovertibly composed of the 'very small'. And secondly, that everything has quantum properties, and we interact with things on the basis of how we choose to 'observe' them. This 'observational' principle applies in the 'macro' world all the time. For example, take a mundane object like an automobile; it can be seen as a device that enables us to travel, a piece of design, a status symbol, a structure or piece of engineering, an ecological threat, an assemblage of materials, metals, plastics, etc., a functioning machine based on the interplay of several interlocking electrical circuits . . . down to the make-up of the materials from which every part is constructed, their molecular, and even their sub-atomic qualities. We see and evaluate what we seek. Likewise, the quantum properties are contained in things that are also subject to Newtonian principles and we 'see' what we choose to engage or attempt to evaluate by virtue of the addition of our conscious observational faculties. Living tissue reacts to forces that are part of our world of time, space and gravity. Its 'informational' properties, however, might be more fully explained in quantum mechanical terms.

Our interaction with these properties of tissue is really to *participate* with them. We find a way of 'resonating' with them as their electrons 'share their data with the observer' in the moment of observation. This lends the whole 'quantum' experience a quality of subjectivity or participation that sits in contrast to the idea of detached and objective information processing in a 'classical' Newtonian sense. And despite the fact that we process all the data 'out there' through our perceptual and cognitive faculties – somewhat subjective anyway – many would claim that this is all we can really 'know'. To conflate knowledge and experience 'as one' has been difficult in a culture that is embarrassed by anything outside the 'known'. But how much more fully might we 'know' if we can find ways to integrate the two through the joint faculties of analysis and participation? In this sense, this really is the age of 'information'; the time to integrate the quality of thought into our concept of reality.

In his book *Pathways of Chance,* the physicist David Peat puts it in this way:

> *Physics of the eighteenth century dealt with the movement and transformation of matter. The nineteenth century introduced the notion that various forms of energy – work, heat, electrical, chemical, biological, etc are mutually interconvertable, transforming one into the other according to the laws of thermodynamics. Then, at the start of the twentieth century, Einstein's formula $E = mc^2$ showed that the mutual transformation of matter and energy was possible. And now, in the twenty-first century, we should perhaps entertain the notion of a triad (matter, energy and information) in place of the duality matter–energy.*
>
> (Peat, 2007)

(At the end of the 19th century, Dr Still had said something rather similar!)

Furthermore, perhaps matter and experience can be several things at the same time, depending not only on whether they are observed but on *how* they are observed: what we 'choose' to look at and what we then call it. Who knows: maybe the 'quantum wave collapse' is a phenomenon that varies according to the *mode* of interaction and the *quality* of observation and cognitive processing. (The role of consciousness here begins to make an arcane subject almost unfathomable). All of this invites the inference that experience may matter more than material fact, and not the other way round!

Red Ray

When I was a boy, a prized possession was a pair of 'Red Ray' goggles that enabled me, and all who owned such marvels, to read encrypted messages written by entangling red and green script that rendered it illegible to all but we goggle owners. We were empowered to get the message as the red-tinted lenses cancelled out the red script to reveal the message written in green. Well, as a boy, this was special, and although the messages rarely contained the secret of life, the principle in the story reflects the fact that we 'see' according to the structure of our perceptual 'tools'.

But it is not only the perceptual apparatus of a species that governs *what* it sees but it is also the significance to survival of what it perceives – its 'meaning' – that filters its impressions and refines its reactions to things in its particular world. To put it simply, our perceptual responses to a mundane object like a chair leg are likely to differ from those of the domestic pet who will not only 'see' it differently but also enjoy the idea of gnawing it. The significance of what we see or experience not only affects *what and how* we see or experience something; it will also modulate what we think or feel we have seen or experienced. Indeed, if reality is 'matter observed' processed by consciousness, the very idea of objectivity would seem to evaporate. Maybe our *experience* of reality is all there is. So our conceptual 'apparatus' is as significant as our perceptual machinery; the physiological and cognitive combine to control exactly what we perceive as well as what we feel about it.

If we add to this the fact that things have meaning in terms of their context or those things with which they are in conjunction or relationship (Stapp, 1971), then clearly the way the observer chooses, includes, excludes and 'edits' this context will also have a bearing on the experience of what is observed and its significance.

So to recap, perhaps we cannot 'know' reality. We can only know what we process through perception, experience, meaning and selected modes of analysis, in part, a process of participation. This often converges for large numbers of observers through culture, genes, conditioning and education to create some broad areas of concordance, but variations obviously do exist: meaning for each of us can vary; experience certainly does, and perception might too . . . In 1938, Einstein wrote:

> 'Physical concepts are free creations of the human mind, and are
> not, however it may seem, uniquely determined by the external
> world.'
>
> (Einstein and Infeld, 1971)

Quantum theory suggests that our subjective experience is, in fact, as *real* as reality gets, and far surpasses what we like to think of as the reality of analysed 'fact'. It constantly throws us back on to the subjective, on to experience as a way of approximating to what's *real*.

Why this matters to osteopathy

The importance of this to our field of osteopathy can hardly be overstated. The totality of cues/clues in the patient both as a patient and as a human being is enormous. They provide a context within which to evaluate the cardinal features that give rise to the patient's problem. The spastic diaphragm may have emotional significance in one patient; may relate to 'patterns of use' (athletes, singers, horn players, for example) in another, or chronic respiratory illness in yet another. In one it might contribute to acid reflux, in another some form of respiratory complication, and in yet another to secondary psoas contraction and back pain. There may or may not be postural significance, post-partum factors (through the powerful influence of the pelvic floor musculature on the diaphragm), or secondary effects of head trauma and the effects of altered function in the intra-cranial membranes on that diaphragm. The extent to which the practitioner is aware of these possibilities will render their diagnostic and treatment approach 'available' in that particular case; it will inform diagnosis and guide treatment. Perceptual 'choices' and the practitioner's *relationship* with what is perceived create the basis on which the patient/practitioner dialogue depends. Recalling Fryette's terminology again, this proscribes the practitioner's relationship with the 'total lesion', a broad concept that encapsulates the patient's 'whole story' reflected in structure. This makes a difference, not least because it makes complex problems accessible and potentially treatable.

Now I know that this is very disquieting to some, especially those who feel safer with diagnostic and treatment methods that are formulaic. However, it is not the result of some eccentric whim that leads me to these assertions. But the principle of patient uniqueness, the individuated expression of clinical dynamics and the immense importance of the human factors that provide context that demand our understanding, these are vital to a truly holistic approach to health care. Practitioners on the other hand access this totality via different facets of the whole; treatments become the individuated expression of the practitioner's *interpretation* of this complexity. Even so, sometimes patients do consult us with relatively simple presentations whose causative elements are easily interpreted without the need to invoke the subtler, more complex features of the patient's history and where a treatment approach might be unanimously agreed.

Many years ago, when grappling with the daunting challenges that this conundrum poses, I sometimes craved the simple straightforward case full of the 'blinking obvious': patient strains thoracic spine – has intercostal pain – receives localised manipulation to release affected structure – pain goes within 24 hours. Or, patient falls downstairs on to sacrum – after initial bruised feeling, patient is left with back and sciatic pain for several weeks – practitioner diagnoses hypomobile lumbosacral segment – mobilises it to restore healthy mobility – pain abates after a day or two.

These cases are not so uncommon . . . thankfully. But many of our challenges are more profound and the wider holistic conception permits a wider applicability of the osteopathic method in the complex case in which there are often multiple interlocking causes producing multiple issues for the patient. In practice, the lack of a positive patient response is often one indication of the need to dig deeper! Meanwhile, if we learn *how* to listen to the body as well as analyse its parts and its mechanisms, we will find guidance as well as method.

INTERPRETING THE MATERIAL

So, this multiplicity of causes and effects has ultimately to be 'read' and interpreted within an osteopathic conceptual framework, and within this framework, there are, as I've suggested, several 'sub-systems' that allow for different methods of interpretation. What's more (and uncomfortable for some) is that within each method, there are, as I've also suggested, variations in interpretation. These variations may contain some areas of accord, but there will often be differences of emphasis and inclusion of detail depending on the individual practitioner. What might be even more disquieting to some is that all such variations in approach can be equally valid and effective (although some might, of course, be deficient, ineffectual or just plain wrong!)

THE EXCHANGE: TO RECAP

The power and potency of the patient/practitioner exchange is potentially enormous and it is interesting to look at this interplay, this 'dance' and to see what fuels it.

Firstly, we have the obvious facts:

1. The patient's need and expectation of help, hopefully supported by a confidence engendered by a trusted referral or recommendation.
2. The expertise of the practitioner and the facility to extend that trust and confidence through the sensitive and professional conduct of the consultation.

But then it becomes more subtle as the practitioner develops a relationship with the patient's 'clinical material' and its representation in 'structure'. As we've discussed, this material is often rather more than the anatomical and physiological detail but may well involve the expression (or not) of emotional and other 'human' layers of experience. The extent to which the individual practitioner is alive and responsive to such detail is partly a matter of experience, understanding (technical and otherwise), empathy, and perhaps most importantly, the way it's all cobbled together to form a 'working pattern' or interpretation that permits a contact to be made that is useful so that a chosen therapeutic model can be selected and applied.

Now the 'dance' takes many forms but in osteopathy it is usually formalised in what we might refer to as the 'treatment approach'. However, as we've seen, within each approach, the individual practitioner will create variations depending on his or her responses to what is perceived and processed, and exactly what *is* perceived or processed will depend on what 'questions' are asked of the body, of the tissues, as we work. The process of treatment is a 'Socratic' dialogue; it really listens as it interprets and responds. And this obtains in all truly osteopathic methods both in the detail of a technique and in the entire treatment process. The connection that is made with the patient is empathic right down to the use of the hands; the empathy breathes with the practitioner and that breath extends to his/her fingertips.

This mode of practice is evidenced in the way the practitioner dwells on certain tissue areas, modulating pressures, rhythmic movements, speed of articulatory movements and leverages during the typical 'GOT'; or the way the exponent of 'SAT' assembles the entire conception of the 'total lesion', distilling it into an energetic focal point in the spine and applying an 'energy-matched' stimulus that in a split second acknowledges, meets and releases the lesion, meeting its mobility characteristics, its tissue quality, and above all, its significance to, and meaning for, the whole-body pattern; a 'pebble on the pond' moment in which the power to reach the 'whole pond' depends on specificity and precision. Or finally, the creation of the 'still leverage fulcrum' that enables the journey through the patient's IVM when the potency of the pattern can be accessed to allow the healing to be realised and the 'breath' to be expressed. As I'll discuss in Chapter 7, this 'fulcrum' is charged with knowledge and both listens and directs; it makes choices! But its choices and direction are born from the assimilation of information acquired through stillness. At this point and to take it even further, I'd say that the conceptual framework favoured by the practitioner almost *draws the lesion into the grasp of the therapeutic method chosen*, both 'defining' and 'placing' the lesion in touch with the corrective approach. The conscious application of principle creates both diagnosis and treatment; both understanding and resolution (potentially). It is a truly participatory process!

All these steps require the 'subjective' involvement of the practitioner, and if that were to be eliminated from our work, our method would lose power; there would be no 'dance'.

TO CONCLUDE: *LOGOS/MYTHOS*

In our dichotomous reality, we awkwardly encompass both *logos* and *mythos*, as the Greeks called them; two vital and complementary perspectives on thinking and knowledge. Karen Armstrong is eloquent on their respective roles:

> Logos *('reason') was the pragmatic mode of thought that enabled people to function effectively in the world. It had, therefore, to correspond accurately to external reality . . .* Logos *was forward-looking, continually on the lookout for new ways of controlling the environment, improving old insights or inventing something fresh.* Logos *was essential for the survival of our species. But it had its limitations: it could not assuage human grief or find ultimate meaning in life's struggles. For that, people turned to* mythos *or 'myth'.*
>
> *Today we live in a society of scientific* logos *and myth has fallen into disrepute. . . . But in the past, myth was not self-indulgent fantasy; rather like* logos, *it helped people to live creatively in our confusing world, though in a different way. . . . Myth has been called a primitive form of psychology.*
>
> (Armstrong, 2009)

In our modern era, we are used to juxtaposing these two qualities, the scientific/analytical on the one hand, the often inexplicable world of experience, faith and transcendent reality on the other; the objective versus the subjective. And here the word *versus* is important since the objective and subjective are used so often as mutually exclusive ways of thinking instead of complementary and mutually supportive modes of thought.

In the light of this, two questions emerge: firstly, why, in our culture, has 'reality' become so identified with *logos* alone? And secondly, if a transcendent reality and experience have so consistently become closely linked with *mythos* as a means of representing them, why ignore its power as a resource, alienating it from the world of applied science (though pure scientists would attest to its importance) and locking it safely away in the realms of art and religion? In osteopathy, many highly skilled (and intuitive) practitioners would claim embarrassment when considering the role of the subjective. It has become our very own elephant in the room.

And already I hear the detractors wailing that the remarrying of these two paradigms is regressive, overturning scientific progress to rely once more on magic, incantation, prayer and the like. But this is a nonsense that ignores how the understanding in science, metaphysics and psychology have developed to allow their fusion to yield greater levels of skill and more complete engagement with human issues, medically and otherwise. Our accumulation of increasing fact and detail always begs more questions, and some of those questions, at least, elicit answers that can only be derived from subjective experience. The 'osteopathic experience' is about human issues, human beings, and its version of the patient's 'reality' has, at best, to involve such a process of integration methodologically if it is going to produce the 'dance' that profoundly connects with therapeutic potential, using skills that are accurately honed to meet the patient's needs within our clinical remit. For, as Eliot says, *there is only the dance* (Eliot, 1944).

REFERENCES:

Armstrong, K, 2009, *The Case for God*, The Bodley Head.
Boyd, W, 2012, *Waiting for Sunrise*, Bloomsbury.
Einstein, A & Infeld, L, 1988, *The Evolution of Physics*, Simon & Schuster.
Eliot, TS, 1944, *Four Quartets*, Faber and Faber.
Heisenberg, W, 1958, *Physics and Philosophy*, Harper Torchbooks.
Herbert, N, 1985, *Quantum Reality*, Anchor Books.
Peat, F D, 2007, *Pathways of Chance*, Pari Publishing.
Popper, K, 1934, *The Logic of Scientific Discovery*, Routledge.
Stapp, H, 1971, *S-Matrix Interpretation of Quantum Theory*, Physical Review, D3, 1303.
Zukav, G, 1979, *The Dancing Wu Li Masters*, Hutchinson.

Chapter 7

The Intelligent Fulcrum: palpation and thought on the move

This chapter is an adaptation of a lecture given in 2006 in London for the Sutherland Cranial College.

Palpation is one of our most valuable tools; the osteopath's scalpel, but one with such receptivity that one would be justified in wondering how it is programmed and what its intelligence comprises. In essence, palpation is as good as the mind of the palpator and it is the creation and training of this skill that is a field of such fascination.

So what do we palpate?

Many inside the profession will have strayed from the world of the Involuntary Mechanism into the slippery world of quantum mechanics and some might have seen a film called *What the Bleep Do We Know!?* – about the 'quantum world'. And because of its relevance to our field, I was tempted to title this chapter 'What the bleep do we palpate?' but thought better of it.

So what do we think happens when we palpate? Do we feel anatomy, do we feel function, anatomy in motion, do we feel fields of function – what exactly do we think we're feeling? The other question is *how* do we feel it, let alone interpret it and make it effective?

Most of what we'll look at here applies to osteopathy in general, but it's the 'cranial' field for which it has particular relevance, and to which much of the material is most readily applied.

The subtitle of this chapter was going to be 'how to read *the patient*, not *the mechanism*', ('mechanism' being a term used a great deal in 'cranial' teaching to describe the embodiment of Sutherland's concept), and I'll expand on this as we go along. Running through this talk are constant references to what Dr Still spoke of as 'Mind' (Still, 1892) – you all remember his triune of Mind, Matter and Motion - and it's Still's concept of Mind in the broadest sense that I'm likely to mention quite often. Some of you will recall, having read Still, that when he used the word 'Celestial', referring to Mind, he was investing consciousness with the quality of spirit. Certainly he spoke about Mind in the sense that we needed to transcend the analytical process – consciousness transcending analytical thought. In some ways, Still anticipated what quantum mechanics might have come to offer us rather later on (in the way that energetic fields enfold the mental process and are accessible to it), and of course there have been copious explorations of the influence on Matter of Mind in some very interesting literature that's come our way in the last twenty years. After reading some of this literature, we begin to glimpse the notion that biological processes seem to reflect a web of information-exchange on a quantum level, including mental processes, and this implies a field within which the mental and the physical do, in fact, interact (McTaggart, 2001).

FIELDS AND ENERGETICS

There have, of course, been various cultural preoccupations with what one might generally term 'energy' over the ages. Five thousand years ago the Indian culture and spiritual tradition talked of *prana*. Three thousand years ago the ancient *qi gong* masters talked about balancing *qi*. Around 500 BC, the Pythagoreans spoke of a universal energy pervading all of nature. In the 1600s, the English physician and philosopher William Gilbert, the father of modern geomagnetism, described the earth's magnetic field. In the 1800s, Mesmer (of considerable interest to Still, of course), examined electromagnetic fields and the way that these fields were mutually influential. Many will have heard of von Reichenbach referring to the 'Odic force' (in the 1840s). In 1911, Walter Kilner spoke about auric fields and the way these related to particular disease states. In 1939 Kirlian pioneered his method of photography which was a means of photographing energy fields around the body. Wilhelm Reich, a contemporary of Freud, spoke in the 1940s, of *orgone*, or the flow of energy that was related to psychic and psychological diseases of various kinds. Harold Saxton Burr carried out extensive research between the 1930s and 1950s leading to his assertion of the 'L' field or 'life' field as a model of a biological blueprint with its predisposition to disease patterns (Burr, 1957). And there have been many other researchers who have researched and developed ways of measuring these fields. A little more recently, in the 1960s, Dr Robert Becker (Becker & Seldon, 1985) made significant studies of the influence of electro-magnetic fields on the healing of bone fractures and piezoelectric properties of tissues. He wrote of the 'direct current control system' whose electrical charge courses through the perineurium, creating fields that change shape and strength with physiological and psychological changes.

Largely through the review of these explorations there evolves the notion that there is a fusion somewhere of the mental (conscious or intentional) and the physical in the expression of these variously conceived fields. Though many cultures lived very happily with this fusion or wholeness as a cultural 'given', it was progressively dissembled by the emergence of what we came to call the 'scientific method' with increasing objectification and the marginalising of conscious participation and subjectivity. However, it is interesting that growing pockets of contemporary science seem to be fostering a kind of convergence again, although forays into the world of 'energetic' fields are still seen by many as regressive. Such divergence of opinion is certainly endemic within our own profession.

To some extent, osteopathy faces a crisis built in part around this; we have an osteopathic 'world' that has been divided over matters of approach. Even in the field of Involuntary Mechanism (IVM) or 'cranial' teaching, we find a subtle but significant divergence between what we'll call the 'biomechanics' and the 'bioenergeticists' and their biodynamic model. It is interesting, I think, that Andrew Taylor Still was able to encompass both the mechanical and energetic qualities in his teaching. He was certainly pragmatic and highly analytical, imploring students and colleagues to dig deeper in their study of anatomy. And yet at the same time, woven into his writing and his ideas was an enormous 'spiritual' quality. He was not a formally religious man – but his sense of the numinous, the spiritual, that actually filtered through his writing was, I think, immensely important and balances his pragmatism in a way that has left the osteopathic world incredibly enriched.

CULTURE AND MECHANISM

The schism I speak of in the profession is both interesting and revealing. In some respects, it forces us to examine more thoroughly what we claim we do in practice. But even more, it exemplifies a deeper cultural divide; one with profound implications. These implications are philosophical, social, political, certainly scientific, and have a very strong bearing on our perception and our interpretations of *reality*.

Our dependence on analytical reductionism has I think alienated us from aspects of reality and aspects of consciousness, even though contemporary science has gone some way towards mitigating this in certain very specific areas, e.g. cybernetics, chaos theory, quantum mechanics and a more thoroughgoing understanding of holism.

In our own area, osteopathy, we still strive to explain what it is that makes us really effective diagnostically and therapeutically. We use tools, we use techniques, we use models, we use information, but we constantly fall short in our attempts to define the complexities and effects of therapeutic touch. Perhaps we need to emulate Still in his ability to yoke the analytical to an abstraction – to a more complete and holistic conception of the body, however incompletely 'known' it inevitably remains. A holistic synthesis is always going to be factually imperfect and therefore has to remain partly conceptual. This inevitably leads to frustration as we try to earn our place in the scientific community, and has led to three trends. The first is an obsession with self-validation: as a profession we naturally attempt to defend as well as explain what we do. Secondly it has led to an over-dependence on pragmatism rather than principle, and thirdly and related to this, it has led to an almost complete undermining of the *subjective* element in the way we practise.

While these trends are largely based contextually in our culture, I want to pose a more searching question: does the cultural view of reality dictate the *way* we perceive and therefore *what* we 'see' when we do? In other words, in osteopathy, does it dictate what we *think* we palpate?

To digress a little, let us look at aspects of our culture, and ponder what we may 'leave out' some of the time. An age of growing pragmatism has seen an explosion, a 'dis-integration' and compartmentalisation of aspects of culture such as science, art and spirituality. They all exist of course but they seem to have become increasingly dissociated from one another.

EMPIRICISM

Five hundred years ago, science and religion co-existed more comfortably; they were philosophically and intellectually intertwined with a shared sense of purpose. Music, painting, philosophy, science, religion, cosmology, mathematics and geometry were interlinked in a way that seems very different from today's trend to separate and specialise. In modern times, science and medicine have been married in a union that is almost inviolable, but the world of the abstract, of direct experience, of the subjective, let alone the spiritual, have become largely alienated and redundant when considering the world of science and medicine. So in the culture of 'conventional' modern-day medicine and science, ill-defined aspects of consciousness have no role. They have been 'superseded' by technology and reason. What happened?

Well, consider for a moment the Greek philosopher Aristarchus, in the third century BC, asserting that the universe was in fact sun-centred. From the 2nd century AD and for centuries after, this notion was eclipsed by the Ptolemaic position that the earth was in fact the centre of the universe with the heavenly planets moving around it in perfect circular orbits. Rather later, in the early 1600s, inspired by the observations of Copernicus and the newly perfected telescope, Galileo resuscitated the idea that the universe was sun-centred. This offended and undermined the perspective and teachings of the Catholic Church, profoundly threatening the social and spiritual order that had been promulgated for centuries, with the Church at its hub. For his pains, as you may know, Galileo was submitted to house arrest for the rest of his life, and was only really formally rehabilitated by Pope Benedict XIV when finally the authorisation of the publication of Galileo's work was allowed in 1741, about a hundred years after he died.

As osteopaths we might warm a little to this eventual triumph over scepticism, but that's not the main point here, for while it did represent the triumph of empiricism over 'belief', when yoked to the Cartesian position that inspired reductionism, this birth of empiricism began to erode the influence of aspects of Mind (in the sense that Still used the term) over observation. Observation, the analysable, preferably the visible, became the touchstone of the scientific method, to dominate the field of human enquiry for the next four hundred years, and consciousness or subjective 'Mind' was relegated, in this sphere at least, to a subordinate role. Indeed, the dominance of 'objectivity' began to make the subjective a virtual irrelevance. However, the culture of reductionist analysis has come at a price.

René Descartes whose influence is so often considered regressive by the 'intuitives' in the alternative world, was in fact a spiritual man whose intention was not to eliminate the spiritual dimension in favour of cold unfeeling science. But in yoking together the growth in empiricism with the desire to see a kind of spiritual harmony that could be based on reason, he hoped to bring to an end the kind of political and religious strife that had led to European conflict and the Thirty Years War (1618–48) that was tearing Europe apart. His ideas began a trend towards the conformation of theological issues to the language and culture of physics and mathematics, and there began the laying of the ground for the enduring debate that has polarised God (or religion) and science ever since, locking them into a dichotomy as false as any. Meanwhile, the establishing of objectivity as the point from which to ask all the important questions has underpinned western culture for the last 400 years, and with it has developed the culture of 'certainty'; the conviction that through rational thought and analysis, answers to all life's questions would be found, and more particularly, that such answers could never be discovered any other way. In the end, Descartes, just like many physicists, realised that there was nothing much about which one could be certain other than one's own existence, hence his renowned *cogito ergo sum:* I think therefore I am. Just about everything else was filtered through our subjective perceptual apparatus and sidestepped any objective reality.

THE COST

So whilst celebrating the essential and powerful contributions of the analytical method to our world, both osteopathic and otherwise, let's consider what they've squeezed out in creating the pragmatic and materialistic world view for the last four hundred years, and whether or not this paradigm has been useful to us in osteopathy and our search for some kind of truth underpinning its discipline. Has it helped us understand what we do?

As a counterweight to this empirical and materialistic paradigm, our dependence on it and its manifestation in science, let's contrast it by looking elsewhere for a moment for some inspiration from the world of art and creativity. Firstly, what value does it contribute to our world view? What use is it? Then let's look at how it's done. Firstly then, what does it do, what value does it serve?

CREATIVITY AND SKILL

Well, historically art has created symbols and images of our natural and spiritual world; it has celebrated power (and those holding and creating it), including wars; it has chronicled events, it has reflected and parodied society. It has also partly through all these, though sometimes not, stimulated us to profound emotion. It has often echoed or mirrored our souls, our suffering, our relationship with nature, our human condition, even our insanity, and it has changed our world view and our responses to so-called reality, both subtly and even more literally (with such things as surrealism, cubism and modernism); and certainly through music and its direct contact with our emotions, it has touched us deeply. It has also held a mirror to our rather infuriating tendency to ask unanswerable questions about ourselves, our world and our predicament.

But importantly here, I also want to look at how it is made, the execution, the creative act and the use of the body and its fusion with Mind to allow for the transduction of an idea, an emotion or complexes of ideas and emotions into art. This involves a profound resonance between the idea or the inspiration and the creative act itself that gives it life, expression and manifestation. It is where craft and inspiration meet. Watch the way a musician moves or even the way that he or she sounds a note, let alone fashions notes into a movement or into a fabric that serves the entire piece. Watch a dancer or a sculptor, watch a potter, or a Chinese water-colourist who can produce an extraordinarily potent expression through the use of a single movement or brushstroke, through the way that the body assimilates a notion and then, almost 'Zen-like', gives birth to it. Consider the resonance that makes a great piece of creation or performance different from a good one. Look at and sense the entrainment between the interpreter and the deep-rooted spark that created the inspiration.

The path from inspiration through composition to execution involves a process of Mind that links to a physical act, a spark, an inspiration, something higher, something amorphous, indefinable. How is this achieved? How does an individual create a meaningful synthesis of something and translate it into a process that communicates through a physical form, through sound, or for us, through a therapeutic resonance? This synthesis is based on the editing and assembling of ingredients that are selected to create intensity and 'focus'; they are chosen as part of the way that craft serves consciousness and fosters a dialogue with it.

Context and the role of 'mind'

Now for osteopaths, synthesis is created by embracing the contextual pattern within which the patient's condition is expressed and on to which a therapeutic method is floated. This allows the view of what we'll call the patient's 'reality', in which we participate by a process of identification or empathy. We gather context in all sorts of subtle ways, perceiving the patient through a series of processes based on our special discipline and everything that that entails. We gather context and detail, but we make the process subjective, participatory; we actually make it interactive, to produce a dialogue that is unique. This is because perception is participatory; it is an interpretation of signs, osteopathic signs, anatomical signs and so on, but it is participatory in respect of what we choose to access and to perceive out of thousands of possible cues and the way we 'read' their interaction. (Our osteopathic discipline certainly narrows the field, but we, as individuals, narrow it further.) This makes for a patient-practitioner dialogue that is unique, and I want to say a little more about what that entails, for it is just this subjectivity that potentises the therapeutic mode. It is, in a sense, a creative act leading to a therapeutic one in which the subjectivity enhances rather than diminishes.

So in osteopathy we create an interpretation by gathering context, a mental exercise of synthesis that firstly respects our knowledge of detail, secondly employs our chosen model, and thirdly requires our identification with the human values and qualities that make the patient what they are. The latter is really a process of empathy which is partly based on who **we** are, and it all begins as we first engage the patient. We then interpret the patient's material holistically and 'osteopathically' (see Chapter 1), as we survey the infinite range of interlocking possibilities that cause the lesion or the lesion pattern to express itself uniquely in that individual. Many inside the profession will probably be aware that, in the 1950s, Fryette coined the term 'total lesion' and I think that what I'm describing is a similar elaboration of the totality to which he was referring. Then, it is the way that we 'hold' this reality, this synthesis, that determines the way we engage and access 'the mechanism'.

LIFE AND MECHANISM

So how does this world of subjective and subtle experience yoke itself to our knowledge and to our method, to form an approach that resonates with the patient as a person instead of a mechanism? This 'mechanism' we speak of is, of course, conceptually enhanced – it is essentially anatomy, anatomy in motion, invested with the 'breath of life' (Sutherland, 1990). It is interpreted through our perspective on 'function' and the remarkable role of the connective tissue matrix and all the other 'structure-function' bonds that make osteopathy what it is; all those fundamentals that our students learn in the first couple of years about the ways that structure and function interrelate. And all of it is conceptually sieved through a model, one such being the model of 'the five phenomena' that Sutherland gave us. This blend 'gives' physiology to the anatomy, gives it fluidity, gives it vitality, and it gives it life.

Vitalism

The mention of vitality, brings us to the concept of vitalism itself and whether this remarkable, rhythmic, oscillatory whole that Still described and Sutherland embellished many years before we knew what we now know about it, has its driving force within the body or not. Vitalism raises a particularly interesting point for osteopaths, though it is of course central to the underpinning of most, if not all, natural therapies. It teaches that life in the material world is manifest as a physical process but emerges as a result of an immaterial impulse. Aristotle was probably the founder of scientific vitalism, and he said the soul is a modality of life energy that keeps the organism alive. It affects the organism without being connected to it in a physical sense. Descartes, the intellectual force that probably led to the switch from Aristotelian metaphysics to the sober, mechanistic, materialistic paradigm of modern mainstream science, altered Aristotle's terminology a little but as a devout Catholic he retained the idea that an organism, being a physical thing, receives direction from a spiritual entity.

For osteopaths, the quest for the origin of the cranial rhythmic impulse is tantalisingly connected to the debate over vitalism. What is it? Where does it come from? We all remember the discourse that used to take place over the validation of the cranial method, when sceptics would assert that ten practitioners examining the same patient would arrive at different diagnoses and different cranial rhythmic impulse rates. The question has to be faced as to whether the cranial rhythmic impulse is actually intrinsically generated, or whether it is transduced by each individual organism from an external source and modulated by the interaction with others, including (and especially) practitioners and those with healing intent.

Vital Science

In this thought-provoking search we can borrow much from some remarkable scientific enquiry of the last thirty years, basically exploring two different avenues: one directing us to the energetic qualities of structural function; the other looking at consciousness and mind–body interactions.

Energetics and communication

As summarised in earlier chapters, James Oschman (2000) has superbly collated some of the remarkable work that elucidates the subtle characteristics of body motion and intrinsic communication systems within the body, and explores mechanisms of the electromagnetic properties of the body itself, its biosphere and beyond. From it we begin to build a notion of the body as an oscillatory, bioelectric, tensegrous structure that participates in a plethora of exchanges with all manner of extrinsic forces, too complex to detail here. Those who are familiar with his work will have read his references to:

- Szent-Györgyi's work on semi-conductors (molecules do not have to touch each other to interact; energy can flow through the electromagnetic field which along with water forms the matrix of life); molecules of the connective tissue matrix are almost all semi-conductors (Szent-Györgyi, 1988).
- Robert Becker's work (mentioned in Chapter 1) on communication via the direct current system in the perineurium, and oscillations of this direct current field which are sensitive to electromagnetic fields.
- Herbert Fröhlich on the way that the living matrix produces coherent, laser-like oscillations that transmit information within organisms and radiate into the environment; these oscillations do not require boundaries at the surface of cell or molecule or organism (Fröhlich, 1988).
- Donald Ingber whose work is very relevant to what we do: his work on tensegrity links to biochemistry: physical forces exerted on the tensegrous molecular scaffolds in the body regulate biochemical pathways involved in determining biological patterns; the concept known as 'mechanotransduction' (Ingber, 1993).
- William Tiller, and his work on the 'particulate and information wave space' and its implications, based on quantum fields, for the role of *intention* in treatment, clearly relevant to any manual therapeutic application (Tiller, 1997). And,
- Rupert Sheldrake, of whom many of you will have heard with his work on morphogenetic fields: patterns of energy which create a kind of blueprint for the electrical organisation and structure of form (Sheldrake, 1981).

'Mind' and the creative fulcrum

Now, if we marry the characteristics of the connective tissue matrix – its unifying function, its oscillatory properties, its role as a communication network, its physiological role in cell function, its bioelectric properties, and its wider relationship to structure – to the concepts that have been lent to us by quantum physics (Ho, 2008) to underscore the notion of interconnectedness, 'participation', and the role of Mind in the context of matter and energy, we get closer to a resonance with some of the embryonic notions expressed originally by Still (his triune of Mind, Matter and Motion), and by Sutherland who enabled us to link 'structure' to a method of healing via the concepts of potency, 'the breath', and its expression through the fluid dimension of the body (Sutherland, 1990). These were inspired if scientifically more innocent or naïve times!

How is touch effective?

But despite all these perspectives on fluid and fields, there remains a gulf between a better understanding of the mechanism which these insights give us, and the 'how' of what we do. In other words, we are still stuck with the question of *how* touch is effective! Meanwhile, the demands of our evidence-based, scientific culture still insist we dispense with some of the best parts of our most valuable tool, aspects of conscious mind – largely because it is hard to quantify or to measure.

I would like to return to a word I used earlier: *entrainment,* and look at the way it may relate to Still's concept of 'Mind'. In *Energy Medicine: The Scientific Basis,* Oschman suggests that the thalamus, which transduces the influence of what are called Schumann resonances (the atmospheric resonance which extends out into the ionosphere), enters what he calls 'free-run periods', which may allow for a patient–practitioner 'connection' or exchange, in which energetic charge transfer can actually take place. He also states that this transfer, this exchange, is qualitatively tempered by what the practitioner's mind holds and by his or her intentions.

Many have spoken about the significance of what is held in the mind whilst carrying out certain procedures, techniques and searches within the patient's body totality (perhaps paralleling the process occurring in creative artists mentioned previously). But I'll go further than this and emphasise that the patient–practitioner dialogue is primed and shaped by the 'human' and the empathic qualities that the practitioner embodies and *brings* to the process, along with two other vital components. The first is the complex synthesis that the practitioner holistically constructs from his or her assimilation of 'context' and the osteopathic interpretation of 'structure'. And the second is something that we'll have to call 'therapeutic mode', for want of a better expression. This mode is shared with healers of all sorts. For those in the 'cranial' field it's arrived at through the blend of the use of what we call *the fulcrum* and the process of visualisation. And it is that blend that allows us to 'travel' through the anatomy supported by our knowledge, our interpretation, our understanding – osteopathic and otherwise – through which we arrive at a point where we *can* read the patient in 'structure', in mobility and motility. I think in this way, we as practitioners hold both the conception of the patient's pattern and its potential to resolve and approximate to a norm. As facilitators, we provide the 'bridge' between the two. Perhaps it is this process of 'Mind' that links the patient's material to an energetic template or 'field' leading to some kind of harmonic interplay between them (an allusion eloquently expressed by Nick Handoll (2000) in *Anatomy of Potency*).

This process or facility invests the fulcrum with massive power, not simply as a potential to connect with the 'eye' of Rollin Becker's 'storm', (see Chapter 2) but also as a hugely potent still leverage point that is positively loaded with information, and directed by the practitioner in the service of clinical ends, whether they be systemic/constitutional or whether they be still points/ resolutions within specific tissues or regions of the body. This direction is prompted by the flow of information that reaches the practitioner, partly as a result of the way the fulcrum is focussed, and partly through the information with which it is 'loaded'. We palpate according to the mental loading that we invest in the fulcrum. Palpation is, in this way, truly creative. We palpate according to what we create as we enter the unique patient–practitioner *dance* which unfolds through the treatment process. The fulcrum is an informed stillness 'on the move'! (In case some might misinterpret this to sound as if we 'create the lesion', it is instead an accessible *interpretation* of the 'lesion' that we create for a therapeutic purpose, not the lesion itself.)

Stillness and entrainment

So how do we employ this stillness, this 'palpatory mantra'? Let's return to 'entrainment' for a moment. What is it? Technically entrainment is considered by physicists to be the *phase-locking* of energetic oscillations between two or more entities, and *phase-locking* is a term usually applied to the co-ordinating of oscillations in electromechanical fields. So how do we *phase-lock*? How do we effect and direct the process of energetic coupling in the patient–practitioner field? Well firstly, it helps to accept the propensity for the interaction of energetic fields between organisms. Then, the practitioner holds a contact with the patient's 'material' in its fullest sense, including clinical detail and its musculoskeletal expression and interactive patterning; and secondly, we 'hold' an almost idealised knowledge or sense of anatomical and functional balance (one that is viable for the patient); and thirdly, through this much-mentioned 'stillness', we 'permit' a 'resonance' to take place. It is the beauty of the concept of the fulcrum that allows us to generate these contacts simultaneously. The lesion, as a focus, 'the eye of the storm', becomes acknowledged first, and is then neutralised or integrated, or simply made redundant. The process evolves from acknowledgment – through change – to entrainment. To entrain the eye of the storm is to entrain or at least invite a resolution of the total lesion – Fryette's 'total lesion' – or to initiate the process, at least.

TO RECAP

The lesion pattern has to be acknowledged in all its significance, both for the patient as an individual and in clinical terms. Our fulcrum, when we learn to use it initially, is probably purely physical in its most rudimentary form. But it becomes a process of 'Mind'; a fulcrum that engages the potency of the focus at the heart of the total lesion, or the physical pattern that contextualises the patient's symptom and its mechanism. The fulcrum allows for the fusion of mentally and physically perceived information within the patient. It is read through qualities of motion or motility (i.e. not only 'quantitative' in terms of movement range). These reside in selected focal points within the lesion pattern that are invited to entrain via the fulcrum to approximate to a norm. The practitioner can occupy the space between the expression of aberrant motion, aberrant quality and the patient's stable equilibrium. (So it is rudimentary for our students to learn about what is normal tissue, what is normal motion, what is normal structure, what is normal function). The mental and palpatory facility that allows this to happen is what we might call 'practitioner software'.

The effectiveness of this process therapeutically depends on what is asked of the mechanism – i.e. where the fulcrum is placed, or the place to which it is mentally directed, and the software with which it is loaded. We palpate as we think. The fingers do indeed think in order to feel, to see and to 'know', to paraphrase Sutherland and Becker.

CONSCIOUS OR INTUITIVE?

Students sometimes ask whether the process of entrainment is necessarily conscious? Could we not merely touch the body in some kind of subliminal state with healing intent, or perhaps hold a conceptual model in our minds, establish a fulcrum and wait to let the body prioritise its corrections? Or might we embrace the diverse qualities that make up the patient as an individual, to 'read' and interpret their lesion pattern more fully, 'sieving' it through our model, so that, as the fulcrum is selectively 'placed', the treatment unfolds. Perhaps this latter is, in the end, where the true skill of treatment lies.

With the foregoing, I've hoped we've moved beyond the realm of the intuitive to a celebration of the faculty that Still called 'Mind' and sometimes referred to as the 'Celestial'. It was for him where 'spirit' entered and empowered the process to play its role in his triune of Mind, Matter and Motion, in the outward manifestation of life and reality. To work with it, Mind has to occupy the place where the whole is greater than the sum of the parts, where the parts have indeed been explored to our best (but always limited) ability. In that place, we yoke the analytical to the creative. It is, perhaps, where science and craft conjoin. In the end, whatever Still called 'Celestial' and whatever others call 'spirit', might be the unfathomable field of consciousness that we sometimes touch in creative, healing moments; moments of mysterious stillness.

REFERENCES

Becker, R & Seldon, G, 1985, *The Body Electric: Electromagnetism and the Foundation of Life*, William Morrow.

Burr, HS, 1957, Bibliography of Harold Saxton Burr, *Yale Journal of Biology and Medicine*, 30 (3).

Fröhlich, H, 1988, *Biological Coherence and Response to External Stimuli*, Springer-Verlag.

Handoll, N, 2000, *Anatomy of Potency*, Osteopathic Supplies Ltd.

Ho, M-W, 2008, *The Rainbow and the Worm*, World Scientific Publishing.

Ingber, D, 1993, Cellular tensegrity: defining new rules of biological design that govern the cytoskeleton, *Journal of Cell Science*, 104:613–627.

McTaggart, L, 2001, *The Field*, Harper Collins.

Oschman, J, 2000, *Energy Medicine*, Churchill Livingstone.

Sheldrake, R, 1981, *A New Science of Life*, Blond & Briggs.

Still, A T, 1892, *The Philosophy and Mechanical Principles of Osteopathy*, repub. 1986, Osteopathic Enterprise, 319.

Sutherland, W G, ed Wales, A, 1990, *Teachings in the Science of Osteopathy*, Sutherland Cranial Teaching Foundation.

Szent-Györgyi, A, 1988, To see what everyone has seen, to think what no one has thought, *Biological Bulletin* 175:191–240.

Tiller, W, 1997, *Science and Human Transformation*, Pavior Publishing.

Chapter 8

The Healing: 'if it comes at all, it comes from within'

Professor Irvin Korr, that great champion of osteopathy, who, as a physiologist, knew osteopathy through and through, wrote: 'the healing, if it comes at all, comes from within'(Korr, 1979). In this, he echoed Dr Still who said: 'to find health should be the object of the doctor. Anyone can find disease.' Whether we look at Sutherland's 'breath of life' ('borrowed' from Genesis 2:7), or his assertion of the body's unerring potency and its drive towards health and self-regulation, the abiding theme is one in which the practitioner's role is viewed as facilitating, enabling the expression of this healing force or potential, a notion common to many holistic therapeutic systems. In truth, the 'liberation' of this power is often immensely complex as the obstructions or impediments to it are frequently multi-layered, multi-faceted. As already stated, herein lies one of the distinguishing features of these healing methods: the specifics of treatment are not in the 'antidotal' agents for disease or symptom as in the allopathic approach; they are in the patient-specific tailoring of this 'liberation' of power, the process that makes the healing 'available'. So conditioned are we to the allopathic model and its fantastically complex and technological basis that the 'alternative' can appear simplistic and unsophisticated; holism almost appearing naïve. However, a little study and a preparedness to alter one's perspective shows that this is untrue and the skills that implement these therapeutic methods have to be honed and developed through many years of study and dedication. In other words, the accessing and liberation of this inner potential is often a complex task.

Many times whilst I have been working with patients, they have commented on the sensations that they experience during treatment. Some will remark on extreme warmth, others will be aware of 'waves of energy' or subtle movement, others speak of a sense of remarkable peace or 'floating' feelings, and many other effects. Some patients say it feels like healing, and some healers who come to us say that's exactly what it is.

Whilst all these sensations and benefits are jolly nice and very probably part of the therapeutic process for some, I explain that, like other therapeutic systems, there is a rationale behind what we do and a discipline that gives rise to all kinds of therapeutic effects but that, in some instances, there must inevitably be a crossover between our work and some purely intuitive methods of 'healing'.

One principle that is common to most of these systems is the *vis medicatrix naturae*, the impetus to heal from within. Whichever force or stimulus is administered to trigger it, the healing is in the evocation of the inner capacity for self-correction, provided impediments to it are identified, reduced or eliminated. (Even for those who might 'prefer' the notion that the healing come from 'elsewhere', the enhancement of the capacity to link with or absorb such healing could be considered therapeutic.) Homeostasis and the complex feedback regulation that is intrinsic to survival is, of course, a feature of living organisms and their tendency towards health. However, any compromise or downgrading of these mechanisms is part of the story of illness and disease.

The science of medicine has been wracked for ever over the fundamentally polarised view over disease causation. In the modern era, Pasteur (1822–1895) was of course hugely influential, largely through his *Germ theory*, in focussing attention on the potential causes of disease from outside the body, largely in the form of microbes of various types. The physician and biologist Antoine Béchamp (1816–1908) on the other hand, whilst somewhat eclipsed by Pasteur, promulgated the notion that it is the body's inner constitutional state that is potentially able to resist microbial invasion by providing a healthy *terrain* that is inhospitable to such organisms. Here, Béchamp echoed Claude Bernard (1813–1878), a physiologist and one of the most exceptional men of science, who was the first to speak of the *milieu interieur*, the balance and constancy of which Walter Cannon (1871–1945) would later call *homeostasis* (Cannon, 1932).

Bernard would hold that 'the tissues . . . are protected . . . by a veritable internal environment which is constituted, in particular, by the fluids circulating in the body' . . . 'The microbe is nothing, the terrain is everything' (Bernard, 1865). It all sounds most 'osteopathic' and the connection between constitutional health and efficient fluid dynamics was, of course, later to be yoked to structural mechanics by A.T. Still. Meanwhile, the importance of self-regulation (in contrast to the primacy of the invading organism) so asserted by these important contributors to medical thinking, has – notwithstanding the complex science of immunology – itself been eclipsed in medical culture, even though Pasteur, in the last moments of his life, is said to have admitted '*le terrain est tout*.' But the linear thinking that is such a part of our culture is much more comfortable with 'a cause produces an effect' than with the multi-layered patterned responses in the body that make the difference between health and disease; and so *germ theory* and the primacy of single causes has prevailed in mainstream medicine to a very large extent. Indeed, people in general are much more comfortable with the notion of definitive causes, preferably in the singular.

SELF-REGULATION

Hundreds of self-regulating feedback devices fill the physiology textbooks and it is hard not to be convinced that many more, including the even more elusive 'mechanism' that creates and sustains life, are just waiting to be discovered and enumerated. Countless laboratories the world over are engaged in attempts to isolate this life-giving force by trying to simulate it. But here it gets mystifying, for not only has it eluded them, but there are many who believe it always will. The idea considered quaint and outmoded by most scientists that there is a 'vital' principle at work that provides life's spark, that ignites 'livingness' and fires the physiology that we *can* understand, was not only believed by great minds of the past; it has not, in fact, been conclusively abandoned and still underpins the philosophies of many in the 'alternative' and complementary fields of medical enquiry along with many others. It also underpins the principle of *vitalism.*

As difficult as it is to solve the problem of what generates life or, as some would call it, the 'life force', one main point of controversy seems to be whether, whatever it is, comes from the inside or the outside. In other words, do we look for the secret of life to an intrinsic function of our physiology or do we look to an external and mysterious gift; a 'force' that we imbibe along with food and oxygen. Well, as ever, controversy strikes, and exactly *where* you wish to land with this conundrum seems to define where you stand on all sorts of issues: to parody the predicament a little, are you a hard-nosed scientifically-minded pragmatist or are you more comfortable in the world of the spirit? The serious point may of course be that these extreme positions are unnecessary as we need here to be open to both the role of analytical thought along with a holistic attitude that allows a role, in principle at least, for much of what we don't and cannot know or define analytically. In a dichotomous sense, we are reminded here of the conflicting perspectives of Luigi Galvani and Alessandro Volta in the late 18th century: was electrical power to be seen as an inherent (God-given) characteristic of living organisms or was it a force created 'from without'? Over the ages, some would answer 'neither', and others, 'both.'

Similarly, in respect of vitality or the life force: can it be said to be generated from within organisms or is it the transduction of a ubiquitous immaterial force that our bodies (and those of all living things) 'burn' like fuel to power the complex machines that we are? And, as such, could the 'machine' be said to be nothing without the fuel itself?

The founder of scientific vitalism, Aristotle, claimed that the organism was sustained by the soul, a modality of 'life energy' that affected the organism without being connected to it in a physical sense.

Even Descartes, who moved beyond the metaphysical towards a mechanistic materialist paradigm, retained the notion of the physical organism being directed by a 'spiritual' entity or force. But the interesting thing to ponder is the extent to which the healing that we all attempt to facilitate or release is brought forth from within or gathered and delivered from without. In a nutshell, does healing treatment 'release' or 'connect'? So what is this vital principle and how does it relate to the healing potential of the individual patient?

Well, it is not inconceivable, I suppose, that both processes are at work, and if that *is* conceivable, it reflects the principle of interconnectedness that some osteopaths like so much. The energetic 'field' that would connect organism to biosphere and biosphere to ecosphere might pose intellectual challenges, but healthy vitality could be said to encapsulate the ability to transduce such universal energetic forces and integrate them in a patterned way to restore the many forms of balance that osteopaths consider useful to health. The trouble is that just as physicists and philosophers have struggled to define 'life', they and the rest of us struggle to understand what this healing essence is. In the end, perhaps it matters less where it comes from, more what the body does with it and just how, as practitioners, we can assist the process. However, if pressed, I think we might get a little closer to the answer with the notion of a ubiquitous field within which certain consolidations and special-isations are manifest . . . like 'us'; and that within that field, a measure of harmony or 'coherence' is conducive to health.

COHERENCE

Meanwhile, contemporary biology might just be forging a precious link between the principle of 'vitalism' and scientific 'energetics'. As stated earlier, Oschman (2000) and Ho (2008) have elaborated the properties of living tissue described by Szent-Györgyi and others – its crystalline lattice conformation and the semi-conductor nature of proteins along with the primacy of electro-magnetic energy as life's driving force.

The very property that makes 'the whole greater than the sum of the parts' in living organisms, the state of 'vitality' and 'health', might be explained in terms of the 'coherent' properties of tissue when its electromagnetic, acoustic, thermal, mechanical and photonic energies are 'aligned' or harmonised. In other words, it is the coherent interaction of the multitudinous properties of living tissue and living systems that create and sustain healthy physiology, immunity and self-regulation.

Now, the vitalists might conjecture that, because these properties of tissue function are not discrete and because the 'interactive' principle extends to the biosphere and ecosphere with which every living system interacts (the energetic matrix of which we are all a part, depending, on this planet anyway, upon solar energy), it is still this 'vital' energy that is transduced, absorbed and assimilated effectively *on account of* this capacity for coherence. Coherence extends to this ecosphere which interacts with our own organisms just as the connective tissue matrix interacts with every cell. Successful coher-ence is the basis for health; when compromised, we have the propensity for health to fail. As we know, ill health can be a product of powerful and noxious extrinsic influences (e.g. trauma, infection, toxicity, emotional stress or pollution of various kinds), or the result of individuated, intrinsic patterns of discord within the structure or function of the person concerned. Either way, in such circumstances, the organism's capacity to exist and interact within its environment becomes overwhelmed.

POTENCY

The term 'potency' in osteopathic thinking is used in connection with both the expression of this intrinsic, individuated expression of vitality, and the accessing and unleashing of this force in the service of a particular therapeutic aim. Rollin Becker was one of the greatest pioneers of this concept and its relevance to the field of osteopathic practice and wrote seminal articles on it in relation to palpation and therapeutics (Becker, 1997).

Like many osteopaths, Becker would use analogies from the natural and mechanical world and several of these have since become part of the osteopathic credo. As I've mentioned in earlier chapters, the most celebrated analogy in relation to 'potency' is the description of 'the eye of the storm' and the manner in which the disturbed pattern of tension, mobility and motility that comprise the 'total lesion state' and its manifestation in the patient's condition, has, at its core, a point of maximum potency that sustains and perpetuates the entire pattern.

When the 'eye' closes or ceases to be, the storm loses power or dissipates. Imagine, in a similar vein, the hub of a spoked wheel and the forces centralised there, without which the wheel could not be formed let alone revolve. Or when your eye tracks the ripples on a pond and you contemplate the gentle force that those ripples carry to the periphery, think of their potency from their point or moment of generation as a pebble penetrates the surface of the water. Similarly, as your mind moves from the rim of a revolving disc towards its centre, the distance travelled with each revolution is less as you move successively towards the centre. At this inconceivable point of 'absolute centre' one might imagine a state of complete inertia, though that point is bound completely and intimately to the kinetic force or energy of the whole disc. It is a point of 'potency' and a point of absolute stillness, a 'still point', at the centre of a dynamic event.

STILLNESS AND THE LESION

The stillness at the heart of the total lesion is, to most, an abstraction. However, its quality must reflect the information that is the alphabet of the lesion pattern, itself an eloquent representation of the patient's personal and clinical material. It is a stillness of almost unimaginable complexity and our means of accessing it are interesting too.

A lesion state can be resolved through a process of acknowledgement. I used sometimes to say that it needs firstly to be given 'permission' to be, along with everything it connotes for the patient. The quality of the lesion can be interpreted in terms of tension, texture and simple and complex motion characteristics. However, its qualities go beyond these, especially as we palpate the relationship between different structural elements and the 'story' they tell us about the patient. These are qualities that require a deeper 'listening' to tissue and to mechanism and they reflect power or potency. The 'lesion state' will reflect a process of adaptation, a coping pattern that, by definition, is a departure from equilibrium. The practitioner 'gathers' this discord in an appraisal and appreciation of the pattern and in so doing, exposes the 'eye' of the storm.

The quality of touch that enables contact with all these elements is achieved through the creation of complete stillness within the palpating practitioner and their palpating hands. And we begin to acquire this ability through the use of a 'fulcrum', a 'knowing' fulcrum.

THE FULCRUM

What is this strange device, and does it only have significance for practitioners of 'cranial osteopathy'? Well it is not so much a device as a method, a means of refining palpatory touch in order to read the tissues' subtle cues. It is usually taught in connection with the IVM or the 'cranial' method, but as I've mentioned earlier, my aim in teaching this discipline was partly to establish the notion of an osteopathic continuum such that the refinement of palpatory touch, so essential for cranial work, would enhance *any* osteopathic work, whatever the flavour. The practitioner's total poise and inner stillness are relevant to the performance of any osteopathic approach.

But back to the fulcrum itself. This fulcrum is in reality a perceptual orientation, but it is taught initially as a physical 'technique'. Typically, the palpating hands use the practitioner's forearms or elbows as fulcra or 'still leverage points' as they are termed in the trade.

These are notional points of absolute stillness that permit the palpating hands to reveal the motion characteristics in the patient's pattern with relative clarity. With experience, this 'device' becomes a mental one that allows equal degrees of palpatory awareness, sensitivity and contact.

The whole concept enlarges to include the notion of a fulcrum point in each and every living structure whose motion is centred on it. In reality, this motion is expressed as an 'energetic' wave but it is palpable to the sensitive trained hand.

THE 'SUTHERLAND FULCRUM'

Sutherland himself based his concept of 'cranial' mobility around his 'five phenomena' as we have seen, one of which relates to the motion expressed throughout the 'reciprocal tension membrane'.

This meningeal or dural network is now viewed as a complex communication system amongst other things, and as such, information is transmitted through it in the form of bioelectric signalling rather than the over-literal notion of mechanical 'pulls and pushes', an unlikely phenomenon that helped fuel criticism from the 'anti-cranial' lobby.

As previously noted, the intracranial portion of this reciprocal tension membrane comprises the two falx membranes (cerebri and cerebelli) and their union with the tentorium cerebelli at the region marked anatomically by the straight sinus which is formed in this union. Many now refer to this area as 'the Sutherland fulcrum', though Sutherland himself never used the term. But practitioners have clearly afforded it with a powerful significance in the reciprocal tension model as a notional and anatomical point through which the entire mechanism can be 'read'. (Sutherland referred to this union as an 'automatic shifting suspended fulcrum' – Sutherland, 1967).

However, every structure and function in the body expresses patterned motion that is organised around an axis or fulcrum. This reflects its embryological development and its earliest expression of motion. Disturbed patterns and the inevitable breakdown in integration that they create not only manifest eccentric fulcra; they reflect the disharmony that we associate with the potential predisposition to ill health.

CONCLUSION

Perhaps we have travelled some distance from the simple principle of the *vis medicatrix naturae,* but it has been important to link the failure of this vital quality of living organisms with functional patterns that can be interpreted in 'structure'. These patterns contain 'energetic' focal points that, when contextualised intelligently, can be released, to permit a strategic, if staged, process of resolution and recovery to enable the restoration of coherence, health and vitality. This phenomenon of resonance can be achieved through that other *fulcrum,* the one by which the practitioner's knowledge and skill are yoked to a quality of informed stillness to marshall the potency of the healing process.

REFERENCES

Becker, R, 1997, *Life in Motion,* ed Brooks, R, Rudra Press.
Bernard, C, 1865, *Introduction à l'Etude de la Médecine Experimentale,* Garnier-Flammarion.
Cannon, W, 1932, *The Wisdom of the Body,* W W Norton & Co.
Ho, M-W, 2008, *The Rainbow and the Worm,* World Scientific Publishing.
Korr, I, 1979, *The Collected Papers of Irvin Korr,* American Academy of Osteopathy.
Oschman, J, 2000, *Energy Medicine,* Churchill Livingstone.
Sutherland, W G, 1967, *Contributions of Thought,* Sutherland Cranial Teaching Foundation.

Chapter 9

Beyond Technique: meeting the 'lesion'

'. ... with an eye made quiet by the power
Of harmony and the deep power of joy,
We see into the life of things.'

William Wordsworth

'Lines written a few miles above Tintern Abbey'

from *Lyrical Ballads*, 1798, London: J & A Arch.

Osteopathy is about 'seeing into the life of things'. It is also a 'language'. Contrasting approaches within osteopathy merely express different sorts of grammar. However, distinctions between them have often created the sense of real conceptual division and incompatibility. Such a position is illusory, its dogmatic assertions, like most dogma, expressing insecurity, self-doubt and self-protection. There is only 'one' osteopathy, though, like many truths, there are different ways to get nearer to it.

Technique

Treatment techniques come in many shapes, sizes and styles. Some involve pressure, others leverages and intricate, ingenious 'positionings'; some employ rhythmic movements or stretches, others the lightest of touches; some others resound with the sound of joint 'cavitation' as high velocity thrust movements are employed. Some of these techniques aim to release restrictions, or to reverse abnormal movement characteristics, or to stretch or articulate contracted, contractured or compressed tissue, or to connect with and release stored 'energy' of whatever origin. Some procedures are 'direct' in their application; some indirect, working with the body's inherent responses that pivot around the strategically placed 'fulcrum' that is the practitioner's touch or input. Some techniques stimulate, some sedate, quieting the neural barrage by harmonising proprioceptive input from different structures related to the spinal segment. There are many rationales and many objectives.

But technique is more than a series of moves; it is informed and guided by principle and diagnosis.

Both diagnostic and treatment technique, at their best, arise out of a poise or 'stillness 'in the practitioner; a stillness that engenders interaction, participation, precision and relevance, a 'dance' that we enter into, whichever treatment method is favoured, and whichever approach we adopt (General Osteopathic Treatment (GOT), Specific Adjusting Technique (SAT), Cranial, etc), and whether we employ articulatory, cranial, functional, joint manipulation (HVLA or high velocity/low amplitude thrust adjustment), muscle energy or any other technique.

Such differences of approach represent different grammatical systems applied to the same language – the language born from the osteopathic 'way of seeing'. One thing remains, however. It is not 'technique' but its application that counts, provided that it initially fulfils certain requirements: it needs to be physically, technically and energetically matched to the patient's clinical picture, tissues and constitution, and it needs to be mastered to a high level of competence in order to work well with these. What is more, and as with many skills, intuitive ability works best when the 'rules' have previously been mastered.

Technique is like a procedural window through which contact is made, intention is communicated, opportunity is realised. It is informed by principle and grows out of diagnosis; it should never be routine, should be minimally invasive and interventionist, and should be entirely tailored to the needs of the situation, the patient's tolerance and the tissues involved. It 'meets' the material in the lesion both energetically and mechanically; it acknowledges its context or greater significance, and it engenders movement and change. In many ways it is virtually *inseparable* from diagnosis. So treatment is about how the energy of the lesion is acknowledged, and how acknowledgement elicits the therapeutic response.

You will notice I refer repeatedly in this text to two points of focus: the one within the patient's pattern, the other within the practitioner and contrived as a methodological procedure. And as stated in Chapter 6 on 'subjectivity', the juxtaposition of these two points of focus is the beginning of the creation of the therapeutic opportunity, with all its subtleties and nuances. Technique serves this objective.

To digress for a moment, there have been many within osteopathy who have felt that all this talk of greater precision and specificity is rather overdone. They often work intuitively to wonderfully good effect. Indeed many of them have developed enough 'tissue feel' to gravitate somewhat unconditionally to areas of fixity or restricted movement and to apply mobilising techniques of some sort with the aim of providing a general loosening to the body structure and a release of tension. While this can often be pleasant and in some cases deliver considerable benefits, it is not necessarily an approach based on holistic osteopathic principles, and whilst it can assist the body in re-setting its own equilibrium, it might not have the penetration or constitutional relevance to move the patient's health forward. The point about working within a holistic conception of the body and applying appropriately delivered therapeutic interventions is that it is more likely to drive a therapeutic process forward both in terms of symptom relief *and* constitutional health, potentially impacting many areas of the patient's capacity for wellbeing. It is not unusual, for example, for patients to comment that treatment has helped them feel immensely improved in general terms, prior to a resolution of symptoms that were their main reason for attending. Indeed, many patients note improvements in symptoms they have omitted to mention to their practitioners.

TECHNIQUE AS OPPOSED TO APPROACH

But next, we need to look at the distinction between 'technique' that is subsumed in the overall treatment (and diagnostic) approach, and the 'approach' itself. For this purpose, it may be easier to deal with 'approaches' first, and the spectrum of these approaches is something we have met in Chapter 5 in examining the evolution of osteopathic thinking that was to incorporate the 'cranial' approach.

The study of and training in osteopathy have increasingly provided more structure, analysis and discipline to the work. A rather amorphous and largely intuitive approach to the business of soothing tissues and mobilising or freeing up joints as performed by many lay folk over centuries has given way to disciplines that have taken such manual procedures, refined and developed them, and steeped them in conceptual models of which osteopathy and chiropractic are just two. The containment of such processes or techniques within intellectual and conceptual frameworks has given them far greater power and versatility, and the greater understanding and relevance provided has produced a precision that has coupled with the all-important human qualities of empathy and compassion to great therapeutic effect.

The inspiration of Still was not merely in the development of such refinement but more especially in the understanding of how this could serve mankind in a holistic and therapeutic way that paralleled and improved on existing medical practice. It drew on an inspiration born from his spiritual, intellectual and medical 'knowledge' and provided it with a firm basis in anatomy.

Over the years, teachers and practitioners in the profession have read and interpreted Still and other pioneers, have rejected some notions, developed others, and have formed diagnostic and treatment methods that have become fashioned into styles and approaches. It is these approaches that have often revealed qualities that have distinguished, and become hallmarks of, the different schools and institutions within the profession. The best of these, whilst not seeking to eliminate the practitioner's sensitivity and intuitive abilities, have promoted certain basic methods whose conceptual basis is to shine through the application of the approach.

My own experience is within the field of UK osteopathy and particularly within the European School of Osteopathy (ESO), though much is held in common with other osteopathy schools both here and abroad.

Though there are many 'techniques' in use by osteopaths, e.g. thrust techniques, soft tissue techniques, 'functional' technique, muscle energy technique, balanced ligamentous tension etc., we shall, as I say, look at the approaches first; and later on, when we consider technique itself, it will be less to analyse them, more to look at the way that, in the best hands, technique dissolves into a subtle and 'energetic' process that speaks of the blend of skill and mental focus.

Approach

Historically our teaching at the ESO has been divided into three basic approaches: GOT or General Osteopathic Treatment (sometimes known as 'body adjustment'), SAT or Specific Adjusting Technique, and Cranial Osteopathy (or IVM: involuntary mechanism, see Chapter 5). (Other technique styles are taught but these are not 'approaches' as such).

If we set Cranial to one side for the moment, the GOT and SAT approaches have for decades polarised students and faculty alike at the ESO (and elsewhere). Interestingly enough, they have both paid respect to the doctrines of the 'spinal mechanics' and mechanical reciprocity, as well as the fundamentals of osteopathy that we all share, and have sat at opposite ends of the same continuum; different but about the same thing, like two sides of a coin.

Cranial osteopathy, whilst on a different *practical* continuum is, as I've been at pains to point out in Chapter 5, entirely compatible on a *conceptual* basis with both GOT and SAT or any other truly osteopathic approach.

But sticking with GOT/SAT for the moment, the concept of adjustment for the ultimate functional reintegration of the body through its structure is a goal common to both methods. Furthermore, they both acknowledge the vitalistic principle, the *vis medicatrix naturae* or the role of treatment in generating the 'healing from within'. However, they provide very different ways of mobilising this potential and this difference could be said to relate to practitioners' contrasting notions of their role.

When discussing the virtues of GOT some years ago, one of my old colleagues and a great exponent of the art would describe treatment as 'moulding clay', and the approximation of the patient's body to an ideal in terms of integrated balance, mobility and our other osteopathic 'objectives'.

SAT proponents, on the other hand, would see the treatment as the precise accessing of the *focus* of the 'total body lesion', the specific release of which would stimulate the body's own complex resolution and reintegration of the structural patterning of the body, with all of the benefits that, through the osteopathic concept, we have come to anticipate at any one stage of the treatment process.

So whilst GOT would seek to 'provide' it from without, SAT attempts to 'pull it out' or release it from within! The leaning towards one or the other approach would reside in the practitioner's mind and, to some extent, in his or her philosophy. Artistically and practically, it is rather like the difference between sculpting and carving where the artist either forms the figure (moulding clay), or releases or exposes the figure from within (the wood or marble).

However, unlike the inert artist's materials, the body is alive and its responses to treatment are central to the process of regaining health and equilibrium. Meanwhile the use of the hands and the subtleties of technique will vary accordingly, leading to differences in both style and application.

Conceptually I sometimes think that SAT sits as a bridge between so-called 'mainstream' and 'cranial' approaches in its mental assessment of, and emphasis on, the biomechanical and bioenergetic focal points in the total lesion.

The use of the hands

The assimilation of the skill, the commitment to purpose, the response to tissue and the information 'held' in its context, these provide a synthesis and the opportunity to execute the skill *in the absence of thought.* Remarkably, as we carry out this skill with any real degree of expertise, it is probably true to say that we don't *know* what we're doing! I mean by this that we are unaware of the ingredients of the process *in the moment* of its being performed. And as with many skills, it is only then that the skill itself can serve its purpose, whether we are making music or health. Although this principle obtains with technique in general, it was with 'positional' adjusting that it originally impressed itself on me when manipulation in three or four planes is often performed simultaneously for the 'atypical' lesion, usually in the upper cervical spine.

All of us remember the process by which various skills in life are acquired; they are built up in layers; these various layers or elements being gradually brought into juxtaposition and then total assimilation; the blend is what produces the product. Expertise comprises the facility to create this assimilation, this seamless union, and to place it in the service of its special purpose. This obtains whether we are driving a car, performing a dive, playing the piano or carrying out an osteopathic treatment. The process that permits this absence of conscious, rational appraisal of the skill itself, (in the moment), is in the mental *preparation* that precedes its execution. Such preparation is in the learning of the elements and the 'how to', and the ability to 'marry' these ingredients to a goal. The goal may be the creation of a beautiful movement, the smooth safe conveyance of a vehicle, the expression of sublime music or the perfect 'energetic' connection with some somatic element that contains all the relevant material pertaining to our patient's 'lesion pattern' (a pattern that 'holds' their illness), and the potential to overcome it.

The human miracle by which this marriage takes place, however simple or complex, is a mystery, but one thing is sure: its explanation does not reside in the elements themselves. Neither do I think its mechanism will be found in the brain. But the synthesis that we create allows a process of *entrainment* to our goal, a goal that is held in our consciousness however simple or complex such a goal may be.

The renowned professor of piano, Tobias Matthay, is known to have said, 'Never sound a note without a distinct musical purpose.' I've often quoted this to students to emphasise the significance of every touch, every contact with the patient, and to suggest that each contact is 'prepared' in relation to a goal or aim that is completely relevant. This will give every touch a delicate poise and a precision that will be 'telling' to the practitioner and sympathetic to the patient. It will allow a connection with the lesion pattern that will begin the therapeutic process through that extraordinary quality of 'acknowledgement', that preliminary process by which we 'meet' the lesion.

This is the dual role of palpation: the therapeutic application of a diagnostic tool, the 'goals' being to 'meet' the total lesion whilst learning more about it. When we come to the treatment process *per se* an 'energetic' matching takes place, either through the use of kinetic energy or through a focus of mental concentration, physically 'realised' through a fulcrum.

So, at the one end of this spectrum, we engage the tissues as we move them with sensitivity and an appreciation of their functional significance: What do they do? What are they supposed to be doing? How are our findings to be interpreted holistically in the clinical context in question? The answers to these questions are made available by our knowledge of anatomy, physiology and the conceptual framework within which we work, and the application of such informed skills obtains whichever corrective manoeuvres we are performing, (soft tissue, 'functional', muscle energy, articulatory or thrust techniques, etc.).

At the other end of the spectrum we have 'cranial' technique which for many years has been described mechanically, largely in terms of anatomical positioning and fluidic, membranous and osseous dynamics. These are useful as teaching guides and as a way of educating the student in this intensely subtle approach. However, the quality of 'movement' involved becomes increasingly 'slight' and the student gradually becomes aware that change follows the visualised 'engagement' of structures as the practitioner selectively and strategically 'attends' via a palpatory process, itself a technique.

We speak in this context of an *entrainment* that takes place; a harmonising and sense of coherence that we often experience as a release in the body. When this process occurs more profoundly, we are frequently aware of a progressive 'stillness' developing in the dynamic field of the tissues, particularly those that are pivotal or 'key' to the lesion pattern or its expression. This stillness feels as though it 'connects' with a deep potency and it is an exquisite moment that, for all its stillness, feels immensely powerful and significant in the context of the patient's process and their entire energetic field. Becker's 'eye of the storm', or the huge energetic potential in the turning tide of the ocean, or the potential held in the unimaginable moment between swings of a pendulum, all these come to mind in the experiencing of this healing moment, and we call it the 'still point': a place in space and a moment in time that defy definition but can be 'known' through experience in the therapeutic event.

Such an event is charged with so much significance in relation to the quality of living tissue and the immense drive in living organisms to express life, to heal, and to repair the relationship with their inner and outer environments. In this sense, we come close to the indefinable sense of an immense and mysterious potency that T.S. Eliot implies in his *Burnt Norton* and the 'still point' of my title.

When we appreciate the bioelectric and oscillatory characteristics of living tissue and their basis in quantum theory, we not only appreciate the extraordinary contact that we make with the energetic communication network that comprises the body, we also get a little closer to a 'mechanism' by which the fusion of knowledge, visualisation and intention creates a pivotal and potent healing tool. Therapeutic touch and its attitudinal ingredients become less abstract and, for those who want it, a little more 'real'. But for all its 'reality', the eliciting, sharing and experience of the 'still point' remain extraordinary moments. Such moments occur in all of osteopathy in all sorts of ways, and the energetic connection made with the patient's lesion pattern in the release of the complex spinal dysfunction through structural adjustment is no less extraordinary.

Once again, this is a notion that may sit uncomfortably in a culture steeped in scientific materialism which is not hospitable to the miraculous, even if that is precisely what every patient really wants! The leading-edge science to which I've referred in previous chapters (and through which a greater understanding of the body is potentially being offered to medicine) creates a little more insight into these phenomena and perhaps the validation of some of our methods. Technique becomes a mere vehicle for an exchange heaving with 'energetic' information that becomes focussed strategically to expedite the most significant move towards greater biological coherence. There are some who feel that this is medicine's future (Dossey, 1982). It is true that many therapeutic procedures have quite definitive aims in terms of tissue change, lesion reversal or release, restoration of mobility, improved mechanical integration, improved neuromuscular patterning, enhanced circulation and so on. However, the means by which such elemental processes are woven holistically into an approach determines the extent to which the functional matrix of the body can be affected in the service of greater constitutional health. This process creates a diagnostic framework and a therapeutic strategy that prioritises certain features and procedures. In any one session, this governs what is included and, perhaps more especially, what is not; for as in many areas of therapeutic endeavour, economy (as well as precision) is of inestimable value.

ATTITUDE

In the service of all this, the importance of *attitude* and *intention* is inescapable. It not only educates and fuels diagnostic and therapeutic technique and the overall approach, it also underpins the relationship between patient and practitioner that acknowledges the patient's issues, validates the patient as a person and modulates every aspect of what is a human exchange placed respectfully at the service of the patient's quest for health.

REFERENCES

Dossey, L, 1982, *Space, Time and Medicine*, Shambhala.

Chapter 10
Placebo and Ritual

Placebo – What's the problem?

Let's just state it at the outset: the placebo 'effect' is an extraordinary thing. Apart from anything else, it is a testament to the obvious fact that mind and body connect and reflect one another. If health is a function of the coherent integration of vital functions, including mento-emotional habitus and experience, the honest and genuine inculcation of optimism and faith within the patient that they can be well is an invaluable tool. If this is 'placebo' I'm for it, since its opposite is the patient's pessimistic identification with the state of 'unwellness', and the impediment to recovery that this so often produces. This concept was not, of course, unknown to the ancient world. Plato, in 380 BC, speaking through King Zamolxis in his play *Charmides* wrote: '*If the head and the body are to be well, you must begin by curing the soul*,' and he opined that the separation of soul and body was the great mistake of the physicians of the time. Perhaps not much has changed in this respect in over two thousand years!

Our physiology is constantly being sustained by mechanisms of which we are largely unconscious and blissfully unaware. Personally I am delighted not to have to worry about regulating my heart rate, metabolising breakfast or peristalsing. These mechanisms are concerned with sustaining physical and physiological balance, cell renewal, immunity and many thousands of life-supporting processes.

Many of these are, however, susceptible to influence by conscious experience, and some are intertwined with unconscious processes; there are countless examples of such mind/body interactions in everyday life, well-known and accepted by everyone. Fear, anxiety, anger or resentment, for example, are frequently associated with the manifestation of so many problems, from gastro-intestinal to cardiovascular to respiratory to musculoskeletal illnesses, or simply with changes in neurohormonal chemistry that will lower a patient's pain threshold, produce inflammation or lower their immunity. On the other hand, the beneficial effects to health of positive states of mind, like optimism, fulfilment, love and contentment are, whilst not guarantees of health and longevity, undeniably significant.

But there are those who take a different view of these 'mind/body' phenomena to use them more cynically as part of a critical perspective on both psychosomatic illness (so often falsely considered to be imaginary) and the claimed successes of holistic medicine, also thought to be imaginary and put down to the 'placebo effect' which, as a dubious explanation, becomes a somewhat overused weapon. Homoeopathy, the sceptics' favourite, provides a wonderful example of incredulity born of flawed analysis and appraisal (if not rank prejudice), where positive outcomes are invariably put down to 'placebo'. (They have yet to explain how this operates in babies, children and animals in whom countless successes have been logged by caring parents, pet owners, farmers, etc.)

The idea that mind and body are chemically and physiologically entwined is not that difficult conceptually; its mechanisms have been elucidated thoroughly. But these mechanisms are highly complex with endless, infinitely variable possibilities enmeshed in complex neuro-endocrine and bioenergetic processes that are hard to predict in any one patient or individual. Meanwhile, if 'placebo' can *contribute* to positive therapeutic outcomes, then I would say, let's have more of it! So let's look at it sensibly for a moment.

Any therapeutic system, practice or practitioner that draws upon the patient's inherent capacity to self-heal has to be on to something important. And any 'therapeutic' system that suppresses it is, by any reckoning and in most circumstances at least, bad medicine.

The placebo effect may be a mystery to science, but this is only because we haven't yet elucidated some of the more extraordinary effects of consciousness on physical processes. But that is not to say that they don't exist or matter.

When a critic of an 'alternative' or unorthodox system of healing uses the phrase 'placebo', it is usually pejorative and is based partly on that other contentious issue: the difficulty of trialing and evidence-gathering in the field of holisitic medicine (see Chapter 3). In any event, I would assert that any system of treatment that ignores the opportunity to enlist the support of the patient's morale and its healing effect is deficient at best (irresponsible at worst) *provided that it is enlisted honestly.*

The crux of this matter may be that when the term 'placebo' is used critically rather than constructively, it is generated by a tendency to divide human function into component parts, rendering a patient's positive attitude irrelevant because it becomes more difficult to assess the efficacy of a treatment process in isolation.

But it is often forgotten that patients *respond* holistically too. The various responses that are deemed physical, psychological, etc. are compartmentalised arbitrarily and artificially. All these responses are interactive and mutually supportive so that any clinical intervention that enhances the patient's belief in their own healing capacity is justified and potentially helpful.

So let's boldly state that use of the term 'placebo' is often a critical device for isolating a mechanism that is in fact part of a naturally integrated and desirable response; an inevitable part of the self-healing on which all the best clinical systems depend. Far from a simple process of self-deception, it attests to the power of positive thought. It has been shown in many research trials (Brooks, 2010) that patients' expectation of help, in whatever therapeutic guise, changes their physiological responses favourably, even when the therapeutic agent is absent. And responses to drugs like diazepam have been found to be positive only if the patient was aware that they were taking it. Patients' bodies retain or regain health as a product of the constructive interplay of systems. The psycho-emotional dimension is part of this interplay. (We are after all immensely mento-emotional beings.) Therefore health is enhanced by its positive expression and diminished by its opposite. The promotion of such a state of mind should be seen as constructive rather than the disingenuous peddling of false hope.

LIMITATIONS: FALSE HOPE

Now it has to be stated that there are limits to this positive scenario in practice and these need to spelled out too. For as important as the potential to 'self-heal' is, along with any therapeutic process that supports and encourages it, it is clearly not the whole story.

Furthermore, the danger of delivering false hope is always unacceptable. Unrealistic and false optimism is rarely ethical in practice. Neither is the notion that treatment need have no rationale or inherent value providing that patients are duped into feeling positive about the proceedings. Such deception has no place in clinical practice either. But the critical appraisal that exclusively puts patients' progress down to placebo is something that any osteopath of experience can refute on a daily basis. To illustrate this let us look at three typical scenarios:

Firstly, on a slightly negative note, not all patients respond well, even some who are fully committed to the treatment process and with whom we have an excellent rapport. On the other hand, some who are highly sceptical and with whom we may feel a rather poor 'connection' often do extremely well with treatment (and later become hugely enthusiastic about treatment, sending all their friends and relatives!) So faith, confidence, expectation and rapport are not of themselves enough, and a lack of these may not ultimately obstruct progress towards a positive outcome.

Secondly, let's take a typical case in practice; a common everyday experience:

- Patient attends with chronic problem of many years' standing, prone, perhaps, to acute exacerbations.
- Practitioner 'reads' the patient's system, diagnosing it in relation to the

patient's history and complaints. Abnormalities are assessed on several relevant parameters based on observed and palpated signs.

- A treatment strategy is formulated and implemented.
- Improvements on said parameters are effected, supported and sustained. They are palpable and observable.
- Patient reports improvement to the point of symptom reduction or eradication.
- This is sustained and evaluated by occasional check-up over a future period.
- Patient may attend many years later for a recurrence or an entirely unrelated matter, expressing no problem in the intervening period. Improved palpable and observable signs (appear to) correlate with the patient's subjective assessment of improvement or resolution.

To claim nothing but the placebo effect in such a case is hardly a logical position to take.

This is a scenario we see many times a day, every day. It's even, in its way, 'evidence-based'! It can certainly be evaluated by a process of deductive reasoning.

Thirdly, the complex or 'difficult' case in which a positive response comes only after the eventual uncovering and treatment of a crucial or cardinal factor; the breakthrough that all practitioners hope for in the tough case. The potential for the placebo response is often wearing thin by this time. Indeed, the patient is often running out of hope, yet the response comes. Placebo? I doubt it.

To conclude, the 'placebo effect', so interesting, so valuable when seen in its positive role, is so often a pejorative label applied by those who wish to denigrate a method about which a prejudice is doggedly held. Given that such a view is based on little appropriate understanding, it is as unfortunate as it is unuseful. So whilst we celebrate it in its positive guise, let us discourage its use as a term of easy criticism.

Ritual

There can be little doubt that the practice of medicine, like so much else, involves the extraordinary ingredient of 'ritual'. It may be pretentious ritual, such as the donning of the arrogant, supercilious attitude that is supposed to convey seniority, authority and expertise (traditionally wrapped up in a three piece suit!); or it may be the use of gadgetry, equipment, gesture or language that fosters the patient's belief that something valuable is about to happen (which of course, it still might).

However, there is a plethora of sincere and modest 'techniques' that all good health professionals employ that are quite clearly intended to facilitate and support a therapeutic process or exchange.

Some of these are about speech and communication and vocal nuances, mode of questioning etc. Others are about appearance and demeanour, all of it honed to convey the air of competence, neutrality, empathy, interest and compassion. Sure enough, these qualities occur in varying degrees and in some cases are all almost entirely absent. But we recognise their worth which is quite evidently separate from but connected with the therapeutic agent: the medicine, the treatment, the advice or whatever.

It is interesting to consider whether the ritual that prepares the patient for the treatment modulates the patient's response to it. It has been shown, for example, that patients' response to morphine is hugely influenced by their expectation of pain relief (Levine & Gordon, 1984).

Few would doubt that having the patient 'on-side' is of potential value. Conversely, a practitioner who is either shabby, unprofessional or simply too unconventional, will in some cases deter the nervous patient or possibly interfere with their commitment and response to the treatment process. Just as placebo effects can be supportive and efficacious, the *nocebo effect* (its opposite, meaning 'I shall harm') might rob the treatment of its full potential, or obstruct its effectiveness altogether.

In a way, the positive rituals or protocols of successful consultations engender a healing response or at least prepare the way for it. They switch on a form of 'placebo effect', a facilitating state of anticipated therapeutic benefit that melds with the compassion and empathy that is so much a part of good practitionership. These are, of course, no substitute for a therapeutic process built on sound theory and rationales, but their value to the process in human terms should not be underestimated.

Many a time, a patient's suffering has been compounded by an attitude of pessimism, the so-called 'worst case scenario' peddled in the name of no-nonsense honesty (or as a hedge against litigation). Much of the time, this represents an exaggeration or complete misdiagnosis of a relatively 'benign' problem, creating unnecessary grief and diminished morale. In this context the 'no holds barred' approach to the risk analysis of certain treatments can seriously reduce a patient's strength, responsiveness and capacity to recover. Chopra's famous account of the case of 'Chitra' is a moving example of this (Chopra, 1989).

The positive interpretation and use of both 'placebo' and ritual in medical practice are second nature to many practitioners in all walks of medical life, but this is by no means universal. A proper understanding and implementation of both qualities is of inestimable benefit to patient care, at the same time dispelling a few myths about the practice of less conventional methods. Once again, we need to be a little more comfortable with the role of 'mind' in the positive aspects of healthcare.

REFERENCES

Brooks, M, 2010, *Thirteen Things That Don't Make Sense*, Profile Books.

Chopra, D, 1989, *Quantum Healing*, Bantam Books, Chapter 1, 11–18.

Levine J D & Gordon N C, 1984, Influence of the method of drug administration on analgesic response, *Nature* 312:755–756.

Chapter 11

R & D, Safety and the 'Evidence' myth

Many of the concepts in this piece have been articulated in other contexts in previous chapters so that some repetition has been inevitable. As stated at the outset, all the ingredients in this 'holographic' subject express their own aspect of a set of principles common to them all.

There have been two major obsessions in schools of osteopathy in recent times: research and safety.

No one would surely argue with these two preoccupations, especially in the field of medicine. However, in my opinion, these obsessions have created a disproportionate amount of concern and energy, largely spent in bad methodology and poor theorising.

Scientific research has grown in intensification and sophistication beyond the imaginings of most ordinary mortals living outside the realms of such things and, for many reasons, this progression has spawned enormous benefits in certain fields.

Unfortunately, in the field with which we are engaged here, the impressive and weighty culture of scientific research throws up a paradigm problem and yet those involved in osteopathic education seem bent on emulating research paradigms that simply don't meet our requirements.

Without dwelling for too long on why this should be, let's just say that osteopathy, like many so-called 'alternative' professions – I hesitate to use the word 'alternative', though that is exactly what osteopathy has been for most of its life – has suffered from a passionate need to prove itself in an attitude of conformity and in a language and method suited to a very different cultural discipline. This is not to say that medical science is irrelevant; far from it. It is simply that our methods and rationales cannot be applied or tested using conventional methodologies. A thoroughgoing understanding of holism explains why this is so and I would refer back to Chapter 3 accordingly.

Safety

Safety is and always should be an indubitable part of practice in any domain. Its status as a criterion of best practice in medicine is born partly out of the fact that medical intervention is chemically or surgically intrusive. This is frequently to miraculous effect, saving life and restoring function. However, such procedures have always raised the issue in medical minds of the risk/benefit ratio, the reason being that such interventions are so powerful and – to some extent – unnatural that they involve uncertain benefits and potentially certain side-effects.

So-called 'natural' methods of intervention combine potentially powerful interventions with comparatively low risk. And this combination is often hard to understand in the light of the culture of mainstream medicine. In other words, it is often thought that if a procedure has the power to heal, it must have an equal power to hurt. On the whole, alternative medical treatments have the potential to succeed well if they are utterly precise and appropriate to the patient's needs and constitution. If not, they are quite likely to be useless, of very temporary effectiveness or purely palliative. Rarely do the methods themselves – with a few important exceptions – have the power to harm. In osteopathy, they are rarely dangerous unless applied with insensitive rigour, over-zealous physical force or, more especially, **they overlook the need for referral or emergency intervention which is irresponsibly unrecognised or ignored**. The importance of clinical medical training cannot therefore be overemphasised in the education of such practitioners.

So if we look at the safety implications and precautionary measures for osteopathic practice, they are, as I see it, the following:

1. The failure to recognise a clinical emergency requiring intervention outside of what the practitioner can provide and necessitating the involvement of the patient's GP or other consultant. This problem potentially faces all healthcare practitioners.
2. The over-zealous application of structural techniques that are either inappropriate, clinically contraindicated, needlessly repetitive or simply too forceful.
3. The type of reactions that occur from unwise or ill-conceived treatment strategies that result in a 'de-compensation' in the patient's mechanical patterns, too rapid a demand for change in the patient's physiological and musculoskeletal organisation and hence an enduring traumatic reaction or unanticipated emergence of symptoms of which the patient has not been warned (so often a part of an otherwise 'healing' process). Often, overtreatment is the culprit here in which interference patterns of response are set up by conflicting demands made in the same session or group of sessions.

This last category probably represents by far the most prevalent and worrying aspect of patients' reactions that raise questions of safety in practice, for thanks to the way osteopathy is now taught, the risks of injudicious manipulation are minimised. Indeed, the manipulative methods taught are ideally so subtle, refined and precise that, subject to the caveats above, the risk element is minimal and many of the techniques employed are at worst ineffectual but also totally unlikely to inflict harm; technique here is more unwise than unsafe. Therefore, the safety issues are largely expressed as the profession's wish to appear responsible, sometimes with an overblown emphasis on the potentially deleterious effects of treatment. These are often based on a stereotypical notion of heavy mechanical manipulation performed on unstable or pathological structures by inept unaware practitioners with little knowledge of anatomy or pathology. Fortunately, these features do not figure in the vast majority of our students or graduates who are, as a rule, both educated and highly aware of their responsibilities to their patients' wellbeing.

Recent articles on the potential dangers of neck manipulation revolve around the possibility of artery dissection following forceful manipulation of the cervical spine. Incidents of this kind among patients of osteopathy are extraordinarily rare and barely reported which, when you consider the number of osteopathic treatments delivered each year, is a gratifying state of affairs. In truth, the way osteopathic high velocity/low amplitude treatment is taught, there is far less motion involved than when a patient rotates the head/neck quickly to look over their shoulder.

Without wishing to sound too negative a note, spinal manipulation that is carried out in orthopaedic departments and amongst 'medical' manipulators is usually of far greater power, force and amplitude, and medical critics might have this 'style' in mind when they caution the public against manipulation in general. If they are wary that such procedures should be carried out by 'non-medical' practitioners, they should, perhaps, be reassured that such techniques are not favoured or taught in schools of osteopathy.

Evidence base

There are many notions that attract an almost religious fervour to establish themselves as undisputed benchmarks that no one questions. In the practice of healthcare, evidence-based medicine is one such shibboleth, a notion based in materialistic culture that assumes that there is only one way to attribute value to any given mode of practice or discipline. The 'evidence base' for medical treatments has evolved largely for the purpose of testing the efficacy and safety of expensive and potentially useful but also potentially foreign or toxic compounds and invasive procedures. This process is based on the implementation of trials that are statistically evaluated and has evolved into the double-blind trial that provides an objective assessment of efficacy that excludes the exclusiveness of the individual in both subject and object, i.e. in both patient and practitioner. The one definitive ingredient that *is* included is the condition or illness under treatment.

As we've seen in Chapter 3 on Holism, this concept flouts just about every aspect of holistic practice and its strengths, and it does so for the following reasons. Firstly, each patient is unique and, as previously stated, expresses many conditions in an individuated fashion, such that our treatment of it is based on a contextualised view of the patient's problem. (In that sense, we primarily treat patients, not conditions.) Secondly, whether we consider that our procedures are standardised or not, practitioners are also individual and have an approach and orientation that creates one of many possible therapeutic approaches to a problem. Thirdly, the notion that a condition is identical in every patient is only helpful if, as in allopathic medicine, the approach is symptom-driven and antidotal. If, on the other hand, it is holistic in essence, it requires a contextualisation of the complaint such that treatment is tailored to the individual if it is to work at all. Such individuated expression of a condition is crucial to consistent effectiveness. (In allopathy it may only be important up to a point, leading to variation in prescription but usually within the same class or range of medications).

These variables make evidence-based research paradigms difficult to apply in such therapeutic methods. Equally, and partly for the same reasons, audit reveals little more than a collation of results reflecting what any given practitioner(s) did with a particular group of patients. Neither practitioner nor patients are representative, and so nothing useful is revealed but the effectiveness or otherwise of the practitioner(s) concerned. It is as useful as trying to prove that a golf swing 'works'; it proves itself in the individual instance and in the individual golfer's hands.

So whereas the accumulation of evidence has obvious value, the evidence-based model is based on a very different medical paradigm from the holistic one. This is not to suggest that those employing holistic methods should be dismissive of any need for fact and explanation; that would be ridiculous. It is a matter of *which* facts are highlighted as being illustrative of the approach.

The established medical paradigm and holistic paradigms are differently constructed:

1. There is in orthodoxy a cultural dependency on material evidence and proof: a 'bottom-up' approach to the formation of notions of reality in which the material, tangible, observable elements take precedence over principle and idea.
2. Linear thinking considers the effects of known variables that are linked and whose relationships are tested.
3. In holistic treatment paradigms, the emphasis on principle and concept as a framework is predicated on the vital fact that the efficacy of treatment is based largely on the patient's responses which are so constitutionally patterned that they can never be completely mapped; i.e. there are always incompletely known variables, and rather important ones at that.

The nature of the interlocking of variables in multifactorial clinical phenomena (which most illness and disease exemplify) is also highly individuated, impossible to fully analyse and quite hard to predict. This is why presenting clinical syndromes are uniquely patterned and expressed. They are also generated and sustained by ephemeral contextual patterns that are highly variable, even unique to the individual patient. It is true that in certain clinical situations there are dominant features – e.g. pathogens and genetic predispositions – but even these are contextualised individually so that constitutional and supportive treatments will need to be individually tailored and not formulaic.

Whereas this 'top-down' approach would then appear to be a distinguishing feature of holistic methods, a 'bottom-up', analytical ingredient creates much useful – even invaluable – information that helps to inform clinical decisions and choices in practice as well as putting necessary flesh on the bones of our conceptual scaffold. So both 'top-down' and 'bottom-up' can and should be married in practice.

PROGRESS

Progress is unlikely to be found in the propulsion of osteopathy into an increasingly evidence-based and conventional paradigm. It resides in the greater understanding of the ground-breaking work that illustrates the complex interaction of systems: quantum theory, the mind–matter dimension, the important insights into structure/function interactions based in neurophysiology, connective tissue dynamics, mechanotransduction etc. and not in the sharper definition of isolated 'fragments' or increasing detail.

Many research endeavours in our profession aim to put on test what we already know (empirically). Others examine the boundaries of established knowledge in order to move our understanding forwards. As practitioners, we know we can formulate an effective approach to some cases of most things. This is proven in daily practice and our patients are our judges. (No profession would survive on a lamentably low success rate – especially one on the fringes of orthodoxy for 100 years). What matters more is to learn more perhaps about why this is so. After all, the completeness of the osteopathic concept has been there from its inception. Development and progress largely involve the exposure and exploration of its mechanisms and their application rather than the rewriting of their truths.

THE LIMITS OF CERTAINTY

In the face of our need to validate our methods, it might be pertinent at this point to reiterate the way that the culture of 'scientism' promotes the notion of *certainty*. Some in our profession would impose a level of critical rigour that is loaded towards the attainment of definitive proof. Meanwhile, as I've implied, the tests this may require might not only be derived from inappropriate methodologies; they may actually be impossible to 'pass' because of it.

For this and other reasons, it could be interesting to look again at the emergence of the scientific age and, not only at the way it has subordinated the subjective mind, but also at the manner in which it has inculcated the belief in certainty. This has also led to the tendency to undermine the 'imprecise' along with ideas and principles that are hitherto unproven or may even remain undemonstrable. But however much there are those who attempt to apply definitive scientific rationales to life, there remain those gifted scientists who are wiser in their understanding of the limits of science. For them, it remains a true quest, where answers merely wait to be supplanted by further and deeper questions. The ephemeral nature of many such answers is put into perspective by Stephen Hawking when he states: 'A scientific theory is just a mathematical model we make to describe our observations' (Hawking, 2002). Karl Popper once described science as 'the art of systematic oversimplification' (Popper, 1934). Richard Feynman (1988), on the other hand, relishes the challenge in describing the awe and mystery of the scientific quest:

> . . . *we turn over each new stone to find unimagined strangeness leading on to more wonderful questions and mysteries . . . a grand adventure!* [And again:] *It is our responsibility as scientists, knowing the great progress which comes from a satisfactory philosophy of ignorance, the great progress of which is the fruit of freedom of thought, to proclaim the value of this freedom; to teach how doubt is not to be feared but welcomed and discussed . . .*
>
> Feynman, 1988)

And famously, Albert Einstein (1949):

> *The most beautiful and profound emotion we can experience is the sensation of the mystical. It is the source of all true science.*

Similarly, life's great imponderables along with many aspects of the 'human condition' are always likely to elude us. This tantalising and frustrating 'fact of life' will always give rise to a struggle between science, philosophy and spirituality respectively as the true repositories of Knowledge. And whereas science or the scientific method and mindset have revealed and produced astonishing feats and benefits, they have also seduced us into the belief that they can answer the unanswerable, despite the modest claims of geniuses like Einstein, Hawking and Feynman. The problem lies with the cultural perception of the role of science and the application of objective pragmatism where it can't always go. Science is a bit like travelling in a convertible with the top down: we experience more of the environment (and the weather) but it doesn't tell us any more about where we're going. In that way, science teaches us more about what we *can* know whilst insinuating even more of what we can't. The boundary between the two is also unknowable, so we keep *doing* science whilst we go on asking the same questions.

The implication of all this, for me, is the necessity to use science where it counts and not place it in contention with the subjective and transcendent aspects of our experience. One must always concede that it is possible to attempt to examine most things from different vantage points. For example, one might experience the ocean by swimming in it, by observing it from a plane or from outer space, by analysing its water in a laboratory, or by reacting with a sense of wonder and awe as one contemplate it in silence. A river may look static from the air, its shape and beauty impressing on us an almost timeless permanence; however wading or fishing in it gives us hugely different impressions and sensory responses. Paradoxically (for some, at least), the role of the subjective has been prized by all great scientists. It is in the field of the applied sciences or *scientism* that the culture has tended to exclude it.

SCIENCE VS GOD

The scientific view has vied with religion in different degrees of proportionality over hundreds of years. Whereas they lived more inseparably 'hand-in-glove' before Descartes, they travelled through a phase in which the rational ideology of Newton remained dependent on the existence of God. And now, long after the entrenching of atheism in modern thinking, we have the 'Dawkins effect' where scientific pragmatism would expunge religion and all notions of a God.

The unfortunate fact is that science, or the application of the scientific method, has become the new idolatry with two crucial results: firstly, as implied above, it has traded in absolutes and promised 'certainty'; and secondly, it has led to the undervaluing and subordination of subjective experience in the practice of health care and clinical skills as well as in the humanities and other aspects of life. In coming to trust it too much, we have come to undervalue our senses, our impressions and the way that they reflect the complex synthesis that is our human, intellectual and empathic response to things. The utter conviction that truth is ultimately reducible to rationally determined elements destroys or at least erodes the value of subjective experience. As for the denigration of anecdotal evidence as a guide to efficacy, I wonder why reports of carefully considered patient responses should be attributed less value than a statistically analysed collation of questionable facts!

As a profession, we must caution against inappropriate forms of evidence-gathering. We need to focus on the 'right' evidence and a method of collating it that 'fits' our therapeutic approach. Failing that, let patient demand and their experiences speak for themselves! But no, as regards standards of professional conduct, that could, of course, never be considered sufficient, and we have a responsibility to evolve useful and appropriate methods of self-evaluation.

So what of R & D?

So where should 'research and development' be taking us? Clearly, as previous chapters would attest, scientific progress in the field of biology, molecular biology and physiology are highly relevant to our field. Meanwhile, many attempts at research *within* osteopathy as a profession fall short in the creation of useful insights that deepen and develop the practice of osteopathy itself.

We can, however, borrow and adopt relevant research from other allied fields, to incorporate their findings into our own conceptual knowledge base. Some of these areas of research have been discussed earlier in this book with the work of Fröhlich, Pischinger, Szent-Györgyi, Ingber, Ho, Becker etc. The insights they lend us expand our notions of what we do. Many of them simply validate the osteopathic method and in that respect don't necessarily change the essence of what we do but confirm that we may have been on the right track after all. For example, the research into mechanotransduction (Ingber, 1997, 2003, 2008) elaborates the 'structure-function' concept revealing, with more complexity than we knew traditionally, that changes in the conformation, responsiveness, shape and function of the body framework has physiological resonances that are profound.

TO CONCLUDE

It is, of course, to be hoped that the profession develops an increased ability to foster and employ its own research; it is after all the mark of any profession that it is self-critical and committed to progress. But hitherto, in its zeal to become respected, it has sometimes implemented research models that have fallen short of demonstrating real efficacy, and some of the features of osteopathic practice that I have outlined in these chapters might go some way towards explaining why. Patient and practitioner sampling imply a standardisation of both therapeutic method and 'disease' manifestation, and as I have expressed, *ad nauseam* perhaps, these cannot be presumed within a true osteopathic paradigm where the *principles* underlying the approach to treatment are, in fact, the only things that are 'constant'. This is why I have wanted to restate these principles so often, as they are the foundations on which every treatment should be built.

REFERENCES

Einstein, A, 1949, The world as I see it, *Forum & Century* 84:193–194.

Feynman, R, 1988, *What Do You Care What People Think?* Norton & Co.

Hawking, S, 2002, *The Theory of Everything: The Origin and Fate of the Universe,* New Millenium Press.

Ingber, D, 1997, Tensegrity: the architectural basis of cellular mechanotransduction, *Annual Review of Physiology* 59:575–599.

Ingber, D, 2003, Cell structure and hierarchical systems biology, *Journal of Cell Science* 116:1157–1173.

Ingber, D, 2008, Tensegrity and mechanotransduction, *Journal of Bodywork & Movement Therapies* 12:198–200.

Popper, K, 1934, *The Logic of Scientific Discovery,* Routledge.

Part 3

Philosophy and the Practitioner

One Practitioner's View

The closing section of the book contains personal views on aspects of life that have influenced my own attempts at patient care. They are not in any sense definitive, nor are they prerequisites for good practice.

As practitioners, all of us are engaged in a process of care and support for our patients, and our attitudes and philosophies inevitably underpin much of our approach to this, not in a didactic sense but as a basis for the humanity and compassion we bring to what we do.

While these things in no way provide a method, they influence our mode of interaction in our empathic role and take many forms depending on our own individual make-up. Whereas our various belief systems should never provide the basis of a proselytising manner, they do, I think, enhance the therapeutic attitude and support that complement our skills.

The remaining chapters contain some perspectives that may or may not be shared, but they do link in practice with our methods and procedures. Above all, they echo Dr Still's notion that life itself is generated and sustained by the melding of the 'Celestial' (the quality of 'mind' or 'spirit') and the 'Terrestrial' (the earthly or physical) from which we derive his triune of 'Mind, matter and motion'.

Chapter 12

The Human Spirit: adaptability, self-correction and survival

The resilience, adaptability and capacity for survival in human beings are, at times as extraordinary as they are mysterious. They are certainly hugely variable from person to person and have enormous relevance to health, immunity, recovery or healing, and patients' responses to and interaction with treatment. In this sense, practitioners are in a 'dialogue' with this remarkable human quality, deficiencies of which can at times seriously limit response and recovery.

In great adversity we often refer to this phenomenon as 'human spirit' and it's something we often recognise very quickly in people/patients, especially when it is absent. Naturally, there is a huge mento-emotional dimension to this, a quality that sustains and bonds with physical reserves and resistance to produce endurance and often survival. This remarkable resilience has been demonstrated by many and was exemplified by psychiatrist, neurologist and existential psychotherapist Viktor Frankl whose own experience in the death camps led him to his form of therapy that placed value on *all* life's experience, including the most sordid and inhuman, as a means of survival and recounted in his most famous book, *Man's Search for Meaning* (1946).

The psycho-emotional element in human physiology, disease and recovery is well documented and its study is well beyond my brief here. But its existence is of inestimable importance to any practice of medicine and, where possible, its support and consideration matter; morale plays a part, so that patient support, empathy and compassion are included in medical practice, not excluded for the sake of objective analysis.

The acknowledgement of this dimension may be an impediment to the pragmatic scientific medical mind's passion for hard fact, but that's life! Human beings are sentient; they live life in the world, not in the lab. They display powerful and important qualities that defy measurement. The art of medicine and healing is essentially a human endeavour albeit one laced with knowledge and learning. Indeed one of my objectives in this book has been to champion the implementation of the 'human' and unquantifiable qualities of clinical practice as a counterweight and complement to the technologically heavy flavour of medicine which, for all its undoubted successes, often strangulates the patient's potential to regain health.

SUPPORT VS DEPENDENCY

Many features play their part in the creation of these remarkable faculties or propensities. Emotion and memory, self-confidence and self-esteem, constitutional resilience, personal and medical histories, and doubtless many other subtle features all have a role. However, the undeniable feature of illness is some kind of vulnerability, and a feature of vulnerability in the clinical context is dependency. This is a feature that exists in many guises and to very variable degrees. And as a feature, it requires careful and sensitive handling. But above all is the fact that the restoration of health involves, where possible, the restoration of autonomy. This involves something often overlooked in all kinds of medical practice, and that is the restoration of the patient's 'faith' in their tissues, in their bodies; the patient's faith in their own health or their ability to be well. Certainly with the enormous proliferation and availability of information, we seem, as a culture, to have been plunged deeper and deeper into a mode of fear and the virtual *expectation* of ill health and disease, whether through what we read, eat, drink or even breathe. In practice then, the careful and gradual 'erosion' of dependency is crucial to genuine recovery and the process involves sensitive judgement.

The result of this process, coupled with the satisfactory treatment of all relevant parameters, not only involves an enhanced capacity for self-correction as a product of the treatment process itself, it also instils an ongoing capacity for the positive self-regulation that we think of as health. The confidence and 'faith' in the self, the belief in the capacity for health over the fear of susceptibility to disease, is a gift, and it is a gift that can, where needed, be made available through diligent patient care.

All treatment situations tend to involve some sort of plea for help, and in this sense the patient abrogates some measure of responsibility for their health to their practitioner. This responsibility is dutifully born by the practitioner as part of the job but it then becomes a matter of judgement and skill as to how the responsibility becomes shared and how it is finally 'handed back' to a patient who regains this faith in the potential to be well.

This 'faith' is a complex matter. Its opposite often involves a sense of violation of a person's sense of wholeness or integrity as parts (or functions) of the body that 'go wrong' are resented or even alienated by the patient. This psychological and 'energetic' exclusion is, of course, detrimental to precisely that wholeness that is ideally required for health and integrity to return. Such a scenario is extraordinarily recounted by the clinical neurologist Oliver Sacks in his book *A Leg to Stand On* (1984), a story based on his own personal experience of traumatic injury and the gradual insight that healing could only begin once the injured limb was 'reclaimed' and its alienated and resented state overcome.

This process of reintegration so often involves the 'return of the part' to the

patient and this frequently requires the prior acknowledgement and acceptance of a situation that is undesirable and sometimes only partly resolvable,
if at all. Diligent treatment frequently promotes this process and the patient
can often be helped to *accept* a problem or situation as a first stage in healing
or overcoming it. Somatic adjustment can sometimes facilitate this process,
though in many cases it precipitates a resurgence or surfacing of stored
emotions and reactions whereupon diligent and sensitive support can help
patients towards an acceptance that releases them from some of the burden.

The 'weaning' process that has then to occur along with the erosion of any
sense of dependency is part of the vital step that leads to the patient's recon-
nection with a sense of self that is whole (enough) and an important feeling
of self-sufficiency.

Now this is quite clearly not always possible. Most obviously, highly
complex, chronic and resistant illnesses and disease states preclude such an
outcome along with terminal disease, of course; while many psychologically
troubled and 'needy' patients can welcome the opportunity to lean heavily
and long-term on their practitioners with virtually no desire to change the
situation or to consider self-sufficiency as an option. In mento-emotional
terms, this might be as good as it gets for some patients though it is a questionable outcome in clinical terms. Having formerly considered this a less
than desirable state of affairs, I now consider that it might, in some instances,
be defensible within strict boundaries, these requiring further skill and clinical
judgement to implement.

THE BASIS OF MORALE

Some of the human qualities to which I've alluded have physical manifestations that are of interest here, and I would mention three very different spheres
of consideration as examples of the interface between human emotion and
the physical. The first is the 'Chakra' system. The second is the area referred
to as the 'biology of emotion' (Pert, 1997), along with the biology of memory
(Hameroff, 1993).

Chakras

The ancient yogic model of Chakra energy is well known to those with an
interest in eastern spiritual traditions, yoga and martial arts. These seven
'centres' are vortices of energy that have specific physical locations, specific
physiological corollaries, and particular personal, emotional, developmental
and spiritual significance. These range through the manifestations of: levels
of self-esteem, security, creativity, self-expression, emotional strength or weak-
ness, levels of anger, frustration and fear, sexual health or suppression, levels
of intuition and, for want of a better phrase, 'inner growth' or development.

This is not, perhaps, the place to itemise and describe these phenomena. There are many texts on the subject and many interpretations of the function of these energetic centres (Smith, 1998). However, there are certain anatomical correspondences with these Chakras that are interesting to those in our field, and although the human qualities like those I mention in this paragraph can, in a sense, be stored in and released from virtually anywhere in the body with sensitive and skilled treatment, certain of these qualities have a tendency to be more concentrated in particular anatomical regions. 'Raw' emotional energy, including trauma, grief and emotional 'depletion' are, in fact 'palpable' in the chest and upper thorax. Fear, terror, anger, anxiety and frustration are frequently manifest in the lower thorax, diaphragm, epigastrium and solar plexus and the centre of our bodies' 'fight/flight' adrenergic mechanism. Such manifestations will express variable palpable findings ranging from heightened volatility/irritability to the sense of 'void', inertia, emptiness or depletion.

Such 'energetic' expressions are part of the interlocking wholeness of body (or human) function and therefore play their role in the dysfunctional patterns that we observe and palpate in the connective tissue and structural matrices and *their* vital role in osteopathic functional terms. The sensitive application of touch in this regard is, virtually by acknowledgement, to access the essence of human function in the respectful facilitation of change, release and sometimes resolution. Similarly, its importance in allowing access to otherwise resistant physical 'lesion' states is of huge value.

Molecules of emotion

Meanwhile, in the 1990s, the neuroscientist and pharmacologist Candace Pert elaborated the interface between the physical body and emotion in several papers that expounded the biological mechanisms of psycho-emotional experience and its manifestation in the physiology. As she says,

> *'our concept of the psychosomatic network envisions memories stored in the body (the subconscious mind) in the form of alterations at receptor molecules which transduce chemical changes into ionic fluxes and thus the propagation of electromagnetic waves throughout the network which joins the nervous system, immune cells, gut, glands, skin etc.'*
>
> (Pert, 1997)

In that sense, all tissues in the body were shown to demonstrate the identical neuropeptide processes that the brain expresses in various emotional states. And as I stated above, it seems that emotion can be stored in, and released from, any part of the body.

Pert's mention of memory here is interesting in connection with the work of anaesthesiologist Stuart Hameroff (Jibu *et al*, 1994) whose work on quantum theories of consciousness involved looking at information storage in tissues. Here, he looked at the sub-neural components of the cytoskeleton, the microtubules, which he states, act as computers. They're made of monomeric subunits – 'tubulin' – which polymerise into microtubules at specific sites. In other words, the tubulin monomers join together to form microtubule polymers. The monomers themselves are polarised and have two ways of fitting into the polymer. Microtubule associated proteins (MAPs) can also attach to the microtubule. Information is then stored by the orientation of the tubulin monomers and by the position of attachment of the MAPs, forming 'information strings'.

Emotion, memory and psychosomatic dynamics may seem a long way off from a theory of consciousness, but some of the foregoing might help in seeing the role of what we think of as the physical body as the repository of consciousness rather than seeing it purely as a function of the brain. Mae-Wan Ho (2008) more than implied that it may reside in the coherent 'network' formed by these sub-molecular units. Given that a theory of consciousness is science's most profound enigma, we can, at least, entertain a vision of the 'body–mind complex' as a vehicle for that other elusive quality, human spirit.

ADAPTATION VS CURE

Very often and in more mundane fashion, patients will sometimes be confronted with a situation in which a problem apparently recedes, with or without treatment, such that they are uncertain as to whether (further) treatment is required at all. On many occasions, patients will comment on this dilemma and ask for clarification, not wishing to turn for help if it's unnecessary.

Patients' symptoms may resolve through either resolution or adaptation. The problem is that, in the short term and in the symptom-free state, it's hard for the patient to tell which of these has occurred, and the problem with adaptation is that it can involve the creation of more complex 'patterns' which can predispose to a recurrence of symptoms or the susceptibility to new ones. At this point, it becomes a potentially more complex situation to treat.

In practice, the prophylactic 'check-up' will often identify such a situation and engage it before it has become too entrenched or established. Otherwise, should the adaptation 'break down', the patient will seek further help. The situation can get clouded when, as is so often the case, patients reserve osteopathy for treatment of their structural problems, so that an adaptation 'break down' that expresses itself in 'non-structural' symptoms might suggest to the patient the need for a different therapeutic approach when the simplest and most expedient way forward might be to follow up their osteopathic treatment. Clear advice honestly given is then useful, should the patient seek it.

Now it could of course be said that life's process is inevitably about adapting and coping and that judicious treatment of one kind or another can support or maintain this faculty. In more severe and chronic cases, this may be the only viable strategy. But the foregoing remarks are more relevant in the acute situation, the caveat being that when some clinicians would maintain that certain conditions (e.g. back pain) are self-limiting, it is often that adaptation has occurred along with the potential complications I've mentioned.

An often amusing concomitant of all this that probably belongs in the 'Placebo' discussion is the patient's remark that, on attending for the appointment, the symptoms seem to have gone away. Here, the capacity for adaptation (or perhaps resolution) has gone up a notch with the expectation or anticipation of help so that things *appear* to be well. And they may be. Conversely, patients' superstition that their symptoms will return should they cancel a booked appointment, is often born out in reality, though fortunately not always! So the patient who 'does not want to be a nuisance' sits at the other end of the dependency spectrum, to be addressed with a different set of clinical skills. (Sometimes this attitude can be simply rationalised as a wish to save the practitioner's time or the patient's expense!)

SUMMARY

The clinical situation is a partnership; one into which the practitioner ideally enters for a limited stay. For patient autonomy is the key to health and it is the conviction, in the patient, that this is possible that is one of the goals of good practitionership.

Strangely, many patients would claim a fervent desire to be well whilst inadvertently concealing an underlying need or propensity for the opposite. Sadly, illness is often 'strategic' while, in other cases, it is paradoxically a person's underlying expectation. In others, it may reflect a struggle for a sense of meaning. Such tendencies may be buried in what we call the 'unconscious'. However, they might also lurk in the complex chemistry and energetics of the tissues themselves where they have the potential to express changes in 'spirit' and morale. Or maybe this is the same thing.

REFERENCES

Frankl, V, 1946, *Man's Search for Meaning*, Beacon Press.
Ho, M-W, 2008, *The Rainbow and the Worm*, World Scientific Publishing.
Jibu, M, Hagan, S, Hameroff, S *et al* Quantum optical coherence in cytoskeletal microtubules: implications for brain function, *Biosystems*, 1994, 32: 95–209
Pert, C, 1997, *The Molecules of Emotion*, Simon & Schuster.
Sacks, O, 1984, *A Leg to Stand On*, Picador.
Smith, F, 1998, *Inner Bridges*, Humanics New Age.

Chapter 13

Divine Chaos: direction, meaning, mystery and the healing state

Our patients' health issues are so often specific manifestations of wider struggles, and even if these struggles are not fundamental to the cause of their problem, patients' responses to them are frequently a powerful part of the constitutional 'context' to which I constantly refer. They constitute the human cement that binds the other clinical ingredients together and warrant our respectful consideration. Some might refer to this cement as 'spirit' or morale which formed the basis of the last chapter, and whereas most people would confirm that we experience and respond to this quality in one another, we might well argue about what exactly it is!

Patients' suffering and pain take many forms and the mechanisms that generate this suffering are also many and varied. One patient may present with a relatively simple challenge: an injury, a tendency to migraine, constipation or hiatus hernia. Another will recount a progressive breakdown in their physical and physiological state consequent on feelings of hopelessness, meaninglessness, futility, lack of focus or concentration, lethargy; and whereas it's all too easy to label this 'depression', the process has to be about more than a label, and the potential for help by which an individual might move through the process towards a better state than experienced before the 'decline' just might be at hand with the right sort of approach and support.

Some might feel it pretentious that any claims to assist in such situations might fall within the osteopathic remit. The unitary nature of mind, body and 'spirit' will either resonate truly for you or not. But my own conviction about this holistic triad is as strong as my awareness of our role in treating it, and I share with many of my colleagues several years of experience of just such cases, along with the efficacy of the osteopathic method in helping these patients find their way forward with the reinstatement of their equilibrium as they regain 'structural' balance. And as they rebuild their 'sense of self', they re-establish even stronger physical integrity that becomes mirrored in their physiology and in their 'function'.

In some instances, the patient is relatively unaware of any physical problem.

However, they are plagued by feelings of self-doubt, conflict, lack of direction or indecisiveness. And whereas I am not proposing psychotherapeutic pretentions for our work, I can vouch for psychotherapeutic effects from what can be a gentle and relatively oblique approach to the somatic correlates of some psycho-emotional dynamics. (Such claims are paralleled by those justifiably held by psychotherapists for the relevance of their work to the assistance of many patients' physical ills).

So, this launches us into the fathomless, irresistible and inescapable realm of 'meaning' and meaningfulness and the search that takes so many forms in us. As I've said earlier, this quest for meaning or purpose is, in varying degrees of complexity, a driving force in most people's lives, and it is closely allied to that other lynchpin of the human condition: the search for security.

Security, meaning and mystery

The 'separation' after birth must be, for most, the primary inculcation of fear and anxiety. Having resided (hopefully) peacefully in the womb for nine months, it is as if after expulsion and cord-cutting severance, a little voice inside us says: 'what did you do that for?' And obliquely or otherwise, we go on asking the same question ever after. The need to solve the problem of insecurity and the quest for meaning both 'drive' our lives and dominate our existence, expressing themselves in multitudinous ways.

With good fortune and reasonable psychodynamic relationships, our early fears are at least partly compensated by good parenting, until adolescence makes waves again as we lurch clumsily toward a version of adulthood (and the prospect of self-sufficiency), and gradually acknowledge that there will be no restitution as we begin to develop strategies to cope.

Many of these relate to ways of buffering ourselves against potential loss through 'image making' and the acquisition of status, wealth, relationships and possessions. Some of our strategies involve a commitment to an ideology; some involve a journey of the spirit or the adherence to a belief system or religion. These are either imbibed through life from the earliest years (through culture, tradition, upbringing or education), or are fervently sought as a hedge against the prime fear of living with 'doubt' and to shore up a sense of purpose. Indeed, more than ever, our culture now embraces a lust for certainty while simultaneously displaying unprecedented levels of scepticism and cynicism. So we yoke this need for certainty to a sense of life's purpose, either for ourselves or for the collective, the human race. Unfortunately, once found, it frequently becomes aggressively asserted in a paradoxical strategy of survival that involves the vigorous imposition of beliefs or ideals and the denigration and alienation of those who do not share them; our 'fellow' human beings. However, I sometimes feel that the atheist argument for getting rid of 'faith' as a means of circumventing conflict and securing peace ignores the propensity of, or even compulsion in, human beings to fight over almost anything they consider divisive, whether it be ideological or material. It is as if, in order to overcome feelings of inadequacy or primal insecurity, the need to overwhelm others becomes paramount and the assertion of 'difference' is the perfect excuse. This rather awkward assertion of individuality or personal importance coexists with a deep need to belong, so that when the total brotherhood of humanity is 'off the menu', tribal factions work pretty well, all too often with tragic social consequences. Many areas of human experience and endeavour exemplify this phenomenon, displaying crises of confidence and fierce competitiveness. (We see a benign version of this in many professions; even in osteopathy!)

Purpose vs Doubt

But returning to 'meaning', I want to look at ' purpose' and 'doubt', and to state a view that some might consider perverse: I'm going to tell you that the former is over-rated and the latter seriously under-rated. And whereas I'm not looking for supporters, I consider it important to grapple with the elusive nature of 'purpose' and the inescapable but invaluable nature of 'doubt'. In this context, I use the word 'doubt' to express 'not-knowingness' or agnosticism, a term most often used in a theological context but I would suggest we embrace its philosophical resonances too. Whereas scientific enquiry would purport to be the means by which we satisfy the need and desire *to know*, our salvation is, in my view, the ability to live with uncertainty and doubt; not scepticism, but a sense of wonder in the face of unfathomable mystery, 'possibility' and potential. As science tells us more and more, it does, perhaps, inform us more about what we don't or *can't* completely know; though it would seem that, in the process, we are undoubtedly acquiring more knowledge all the time. The greatest scientific minds know this, of course. Einstein himself said: 'The most beautiful and profound emotion we can experience is the sensation of the mystical . . . it is the source of all true science . . .' (Einstein, 1949).

And the physicist Richard Feynman referred to science as 'the satisfactory philosophy of ignorance'. He writes:

> *'With more knowledge comes a deeper, more wonderful mystery, luring one on to penetrate deeper still. Never concerned that the answer may prove disappointing, with pleasure and confidence we turn over each new stone to find unimagined strangeness leading on to more wonderful questions and mysteries . . .'*
>
> (Feynman, 1988)

Meanwhile, I often think it's hard not to be impressed by just how 'unknowing' we are about most things! It's difficult to ignore the enormous breadth and depth of information and knowledge out there in the world. Yet it's probably true to say that, in the main, most of us know very little about anything, excepting perhaps our own particular fields of endeavour and those things closest to our own personal spheres. Even then, the wisest people I've ever known claim to know nothing very much at all! And yet for many, we orientate ourselves in our world by convincing ourselves we know more than we do, and so we hold strident opinions on everything from economics to politics, psychology, religion, philosophy, art, anything at all. Indeed, it is often felt that not to have an opinion on such things is spineless and weak, so we often make passionate assertions about important things from a position of almost total ignorance. And to be passionate is considered more worthy than to be uncertain or equivocate. Rowan Williams once stated ruefully and with typical wisdom that, on becoming Archbishop of Canterbury, he became aware that it was no longer acceptable to see 'both sides of the argument'!

Our assumptions are that life's big questions are answerable, as if truth always resides at one end of a spectrum of argument or the other. Perhaps we should, at least, acknowledge the fact that the opinions that we consider objective and definitive are, in fact, highly subjective, personal perspectives. I prefer to think that 'truths' are often concealed, enfolded in a matrix whose boundaries may in part comprise extremes of viewpoint or argument. The extremes themselves reflect a solipsistic view, the products of our own needs, prejudices and experiences. So much for certainty!

TRANSCENDENCE

Human beings have the supreme ability to respond to the need for hope, transcendence, immortality or just something better. They encapsulate this in ritual, religion, spiritual practices, artefacts, buildings, art and music and imbue these things with a transcendent quality that they themselves (humankind) have produced. In so doing they often create incredible beauty, albeit as a testament to, or in honour of, an indefinable transcendent quality crystallised in these forms, man-made though 'spiritually' inspired.

These testaments to a higher 'power' are the creation of the human spirit in all its hopeful glory. It is often manifest in the most wonderful of human achievements. For example, great cities that encapsulate the fusion of art, civilisation, beauty and religious and cultural tradition; they lock into being manifestations of the highest ideals that support a sense of the permanence of all that is fine and hopeful about human existence. In this way they provide human beings with a foundation, an enduring sense of security in a changing and challenging world.

But the question remains: is this 'spirit', in a dualistic sense, the expression of an extrinsic power that has its origins in something or somewhere else? In other words, is it driven or generated by something external? Can it be differentiated from that other mystery, 'consciousness' with its unfathomable resonances with the universal 'unknown'? Well, whichever way one finds to answer these questions, there is a response which holds power and value. It is an undisputed (maybe I should say oft disputed!) fact that the subordination of ego and 'self' to the *notion* of something 'higher' or 'other' is a principle that affords great benefit. For many, the externalisation – if not deification – of this 'something' is important and powerful. For others, a 'non-dualistic' principle, an 'immanence' or 'god residing within', is more comfortable. And then for others still, it may simply be the profound acceptance of the awe-inspiring complexity of life that gently eases the ego-self into a position of respectful subordination to the 'God' that cannot be 'named', that cannot be 'known' (or to no god at all). To live with this notion in whichever form is the seed of humility and the basis of compassion (though for some, this idea may, of course, remain enigmatic or even irrelevant).

But whichever way works for the individual, the *definition* of 'god' is as futile as it is unnecessary (along with the battles fought in its cause). For it is the 'surrender of self' that creates value and not the *object* of the surrender itself. It is devotional and unconditional in the sense that its *object* cannot be defined. In this respect, the tendency to anthropomorphise God has been problematic, and to infer by over-literal interpretation that man is made in God's image is surely to 'debase the currency'. Instead perhaps it is a call to a state of being to which the human spirit might aspire.

So human beings create great beauty. Perhaps they create it (rather than channel it) in the same miraculous way that aeroplanes defy gravity and fly. The property of flight is not 'breathed' into aeroplanes; they are formed that way. Part of the wonder of humanity is that it can 'create', for whatever lofty purpose. And here resides the dilemma: is such loftiness a reflection of our need and the product of our creativity, or is it the conscious or unconscious transduction of a universal or 'divine' force that works through us? Whichever, this creative impulse and its inspiration form an extraordinary phenomenon, and many of us have seen parallels with the concept of *vitalism* and its life-sustaining role, a role that lends power or potency to the work of healing that we attempt to express.

Healing and the patient's reality

Returning to science, doubt, and oft derided *vitalism*, it is, perhaps, the educated and informed position of 'doubt' that both engenders a healing state that can also access the patient's 'reality'. However much our therapeutic discipline is structured, however complex its rules and protocols, there is something in the stance of 'not knowing' that couples with the stillness created in the therapeutic moment that engenders change. This calls to mind philosopher Martin Heidegger's *primordial thinking; the listening receptive attitude characterised by silence* (Heidegger, 1976); not so much an active process of logic but something that revealed itself within us (Armstrong, 2009).

Though it is not a comfortable assertion to make in a contemporary medical context, the foregoing represents an attempt to survive the polarisation of 'head and heart' that was a product of Enlightenment values when "[we see] the culmination of a vision based on Galileo's mechanistic science, Descartes' quest for autonomous certainty and Newton's cosmic laws . . . Reason was the only path to truth . . ." (Armstrong, 2009). But for all of them, their rational ideology was entirely dependent upon the existence of God, thus 'head' and 'heart' were polarised but both acknowledged. There was a role for *mythos* **and** *logos*; they were not mutually exclusive as they have become in the culture of today.

The role that religion continued to play during the development of this dominance of rationality might seem perplexing now when we *are* accustomed to polarising science and spirituality to the point of mutual exclusivity. However, although in the 'modern' era such a situation obtains, the transformational properties of ritual and symbol cannot be denied. I would suggest that many a confirmed atheist would admit to being emotionally moved by many of the works of creation inspired by religion and spirituality: music, art, architecture, along with the effects of powerful common experience when amongst worshippers sharing ritual moments.

The fact that we struggle to define this response is *precisely* what gives such experience its transcendent quality and value, and I would suggest that in such experience we move closer to a way of being that subverts or subordinates the ego-self making it less dominant; it is moved gently but powerfully to the periphery and in some instances is excluded completely.

The humble practitioner

The point of this exploration is that, in the most potent therapeutic events, whether it is the accuracy and clarity of the diagnostic process or the exquisite quality of the best treatments, the absence of ratiocination that occurs in this 'egoless' realm represents a parallel to the transcendent quality to which I refer.

This humble position is echoed in the view famously expressed by Rollin Becker in his seminal articles on Palpation (Becker, 1963) in which he describes the three 'diagnostic interpretations' of the patient's condition:

1. The patient's view of what's wrong with them.
2. The practitioner's informed and educated view.
3. The patient's own body's certain *knowledge* of exactly what the problem is.

From this, Becker entreats us to value the first two, but to develop a profound listening respect for number 3, so that, paralleling our respect for the patient's feelings and our own educated assessment, we cultivate the means to listen to and interpret the patient's body from which our diagnosis is truly, if sometimes wordlessly, refined.

Whilst the skilled practitioner is, of course, armed with knowledge, understanding and technical ability, there is a part of him/her that can transcend objective certainty and, through complex subjective reactions and responses, link with that selfless humility that empowers the therapeutic event. It is, in effect, a partial surrender that follows a complete assimilation of all relevant material, including the elements of the therapeutic manoeuvre itself. In this respect there is some common ground with many other skills, whether high-board diving, martial arts, throwing pots or playing music. In our own field the fundamental fact that the work is dependent on skill and skilful execution makes the foregoing important. There is, in other words, a quantum leap between the rational process of analysis and analytical deduction (with the assimilation of detail) on the one hand, and its 'translation' into the 'dance' that produces the refined qualities of treatment on the other. Here, the 'science' and the 'art' of the work conjoin. The assimilation of fact and detail melts into a synthesis that is devoid of judgement, dogma or 'ego', and because of this, becomes even more imbued with possibility and potential.

Now, while many might hesitate to draw such parallels between aspects of practitionership and the 'spiritual' – something that will be comfortable for some but anathema to others – there are, as I have tried to express, certain common threads.

TO RECAP

So-called 'spiritual' experience removes what I'll call our psychic and psychological 'centre' from within and directs it towards a *something* or a *somewhere* else. In the wider world, something powerful happens when we experience this, whether in the name of a deity, a religion, a spiritual path or journey or some other belief system. The agent of what I'll call *transcendence* may not be the 'god', 'the path' or any other kind of entity. (Such a conception can become almost idolatrous in its limited definition, after all.) But it is perhaps more like a process by which we create the notion of, connection with, and reverence for, a unifying principle that is not solipsistic and not intrinsic to ourselves. It is a form of *surrender*.

Religion often provides embellishment and facilitation in this regard through intensification though, simplistically, it could be said, it has often achieved it patronisingly through dogma and the inculcation of fear rather than reverence. The uniting of adherents or devotees to any ideology can, and often does, become exclusivist and intolerant at which point it becomes not so much spiritual or religious but political. On the other hand, there is no denying the fact that symbol and collective ritual experience can do two important things: firstly, they can render the ineffable in some sense 'attainable'. And secondly, they can 'lubricate' the process of transcendence or surrender. When this becomes institutionalised, as it inevitably does, it can become very powerful indeed, though sadly its spiritual purpose sometimes becomes blurred, dogmatic and distorted.

The diminution of the ego to a 'participatory' role can truly engender a sense of unity, sharing and mutuality that overcomes the 'self' to give way to a process of identification, empathy and what was encapsulated in Confucius' Golden Rule: what you do not wish for yourself, do not do to others (or do unto others as you would have them do unto you): compassion. Self-respect here is never trumped by self-righteousness.

SO BACK TO HEALTH CARE

Such qualities of understanding, identification, empathy, respect and compassion will readily be recognised as fundamental to the practice of any health-care discipline and the profound 'vision' that they can incorporate. But without them, the transition from a summation of 'facts' to a workable holistic diagnosis and an effective treatment strategy becomes harder, sometimes impossible.

For me then, transcendence and the subordination of the 'ego state' are engendered by, if not dependent upon, a somewhat rarefied state of wonder that carries with it a measure of *doubt* and *uncertainty*. In other words, it is doubt, uncertainty and the profound *acceptance* of our primal insecurity that make transcendence possible. In religious and spiritual practice, this may come about through the way that the perplexing and unfathomable are made accessible through myth, symbol and ritual, while at the same time the perpetuation of mystery has its place, as if the certainty of dogma would 'burst the balloon' of faith. Here the paradox lies in the inescapable fact that human beings are desperate for certainty – to the extent, as I've said, that they have gone to war countless times in the defence of their various interpretations of it – and yet their very hope, their very salvation is, in my view, exquisitely enfolded in its opposite.

Likewise, the struggle over the need for 'purpose', either as individuals or for creation as a whole, has always exercised our minds. In the end, there are perhaps three positions on this: firstly the conviction that life has a purpose and that it is graspable; second, that life has a purpose but who knows (God knows?), what it is; and thirdly, that a purpose-driven interpretation of life is inaccessible or wholly denied. Of this last category there are two further sub-divisions: the first leads to distress or despair; the second is celebratory at the enhanced sense of wonder and the business of being alive. Here, I am contrasting living in uncertainty *without* fear, as opposed to living in uncertainty *with* it. At this point, I can't resist borrowing from *The Immortality Commission* by John Gray (2011) in which he quotes the writer Richard Jefferies (1848–1887) whose first novel was published in 1874, the year Still gave us osteopathy:

> 'When at last I had disabused my mind of the enormous imposture of a design, an object, and an end, a purpose and a system, I began to see dimly how much more grandeur, beauty and hope there is in a divine chaos – not chaos in the sense of disorder or confusion, but simply the absence of order – than there is in a universe made by pattern . . . Logically, that which has a design or a purpose has a limit. The very idea of a design or purpose has grown repulsive to me on account of its littleness. I do not venture, for a moment, even to attempt to supply a reason to take the place of the exploded plan . . . I look at the sunshine, and feel that there is no contracted order: there is divine chaos, and, in it, limitless hope and possibilities
>
> (Jefferies, 1983).'

And as we let go of the obsession with certainty to embrace the potential and unfathomable complexity of living, we might just taste wonder, liberation and, as Jefferies says, hope.

TO CONCLUDE

For us as practitioners, the sense of this special kind of doubt may ultimately be a blessing. Through it we can truly share in what it is to be human with every patient. It teaches us a humility, a position of non-judgement, that enables the 'stillness' we require to practise with clarity, and to develop the facility to resonate with the patient's process without being able to define it completely. For some, this parallels the spiritual resonance with the god that more especially defies definition. It is the doubt that makes transcendence possible, rendering the scientific pragmatism/spirituality debate little more than a false dichotomy and, therefore, pointless. The subjective element that I have been at pains to promote is not a matter of subjective judgement. It is a non-judging position that permits a fusion in the practitioner's mind of all related ingredients in the complex 'total lesion' presentation that the patient brings. It is the opposite of 'dogma', that impediment to the capacity to be open to infinite possibility – whether in life or in the 'lesion'. Only then can the *entrainment* take place and the healing occur.

As an attitude, this places us in a position of submission to a set of principles or a model. And this stands parallel to the prevailing reductionist culture of the science of the modern era. When we consider the increasing complexity of our world, its globalisation, its increasing population and the rising insecurity that all this brings, it is perhaps inevitable that we should wish to depend more and more on methods and protocols that provide 'certainty' and control. The 'scientific method' that is traditionally reductionist fits these needs perfectly.

But our modern era has also seen the birth and growth of systems theory, chaos theory, quantum theory and holism. These insinuate a distinct problem with certainty. With them, we are in the realms of interaction, interconnectedness, infinite variability, uncertainty, randomness, probability and the lack of definitive knowledge of *all* possible ingredients in any system, organism, or phenomenon. We are, in other words, thrown back on to a dependency on our 'model', which acknowledges a limit to what can be 'known' at any one time but which furnishes us with a 'map' with which to negotiate the terrain.

The reductionism of the last 400 years has enabled and continues to enable us to 'do our best' with the perceived totality of what is known to date. And as we know, though so often remarkable, the products of such endeavours are usually superseded as time goes by, radically revolutionising our views and understanding in the name of progress. It is well known that several eminent scientists at the turn of the 19th and 20th centuries believed that science, based on Newtonian principles, had virtually completed its task in explaining reality, our existence and the cosmos, but for a few i's to be dotted and t's to be crossed. And thereupon, quantum mechanics was born and completely overturned that view for ever. As we know, science is still in search of what is considered to be the elusive unifying link between classical Newtonian physics, relativity theory and quantum mechanics, and this will deposit another paradigm in our laps to trigger more intellectual forays on our 'journey without end'.

Strangely perhaps, it is the models such as holism that endure. They stay with us as principles, *with* all the gaps in knowledge that they attempt to bridge, and their overarching concepts provide us with 'method' which is surprisingly durable and, as methods go, surprisingly safe. And while it is wonderful to insert more pieces of the puzzle to support the models we use, the fundamentals of the model don't really change; the theories and methods they sustain simply get richer. It's those gaps, those 'spaces' again that, for all their indeterminacy, hold the key to understanding; understanding without complete 'definition'. In some forms of health care that provides the opportunity to place the technical at the service of the empathic and compassionate side of healing.

REFERENCES:

Armstrong, K, 2009, *The Case for God*, The Bodley Head.

Becker, R, 1963, Diagnostic touch: its principles and application. In: *Academy of Applied Osteopathy Year Book*.

Einstein, A, 1949, The World as I see it, *Forum & Century* 84: 193–194.

Feynman, R, 1988, *What Do You Care What Other People Think?* Norton & Co.

Gray, J, 2011, *The Immortality Commission*, Allen Lane.

Heidegger, M, 1976, Only a god can save us, *Der Spiegel* (vol 30, no 23).

Jefferies, R, 1983, Absence of design in nature, *Landscape with Figures*, Penguin.

Chapter 14

The exquisite nature of Paradox

'For whoever wills to save his soul destroys it but whoever will give up his soul for my sake, this one saves it.'

Luke 9:24

A paradox is a statement or notion that appears to contain two or more contradictory truths. There are so many examples of this in life. Perhaps the most significant relates to the material in the last chapter regarding the human need for, and obsession with, certainty whilst our *real* security and 'salvation' lie in the complete acceptance of its opposite.

Alan Watts' preface to his *The Wisdom of Insecurity* (1951) opens with his reference to the 'law of reversed effort'; another example that we see played out in many aspects of our lives:

'When you try to stay on the surface of water, you sink; but when you try to sink you float. When you hold your breath you lose it – which immediately calls to mind an ancient and much neglected saying, "whosoever would save his soul shall lose it."'

Whether actively pursuing happiness or anything profound, we see here the ubiquitous life paradox: the futility of striving when striving overwhelms the ability to simply *be* in and with our experience.

PARADOX BREEDING CONFLICT

The word 'paradox' is a term sometimes used inaccurately to mean *contradiction* and we've met many of those, just in the controversial world of osteopathy. Individual practitioners have often expressed the exclusivity and superiority of a particular approach, even to the extent of denigrating others' ideas, while, paradoxically, their ideas are reducible to the same basic aims and principles. In fact, some of the more pragmatic operators with little time for the subtle and the 'energy-based' concepts in our work do in fact display precisely those subtle qualities in the complex expertise that they demonstrate every day. Paradoxically, their skills and their hands contain what their analytical minds might not.

Meanwhile, the devastating, wasteful and destructive impact of the conflict between religious and political factions is well-known to everyone. What makes the word 'paradox' interesting in this context is the fact that, at their true and fundamental roots, most opinionated 'groups' in any field have aims and aspirations that do, in fact, converge, though they may have different ideas about reaching them. The 'paradox' that manifests so often reflects falsely dichotomous views based more on social, tribal and psychological needs rather than the inherent content of the 'message' itself. In this respect many with strident views simply camouflage their own feelings of insecurity to foster a more dominant position, and it is here, perhaps, that we see the difference between living *with* uncertainty and living in fear of it; so those of an extreme or 'fundamentalist' mentality cannot celebrate difference but deconstruct it through bold assertion, rejection and even hatred.

But paradox is about *apparent* contradiction and, by its very existence, will often have an undiscovered truth enfolded or even concealed within it. And as already said, we encounter a prime example when grappling with our obsession with the articulation of the ineffable. Now whereas this might appear to be a formula for hopelessness, I would assert that it is precisely this situation in which truth may be concealed. Furthermore, it can be the unfathomable conflict of *apparent* opposites (and the illusion of incompatibility) that creates the tussle that drives creative imagination and life's dynamic thrust.

It is often said, cynically perhaps, that if a tabloid journalist can't get the story they're after, they'll make it up. And it is a feature of our 'human condition' that our lust for fact and certainty and their somewhat elusive nature leads mankind to create or formulate them. Once they are created, we, as a species, will go to almost any lengths to assert and protect our version of them – even to the extent of wholesale annihilation of detractors. We desperately seek to explain the inexplicable and then to rationalise our position politically, socially or 'spiritually'.

Bizarrely, at its extreme, the 'brotherhood of man' engages collectively and insanely in the contriving of life's antithesis (often through genocide) in order to assert a sense of its meaning. At its most stark, it sometimes seems that in a collective sense, there is a primitive but camouflaged commitment to the idea that only through death can we 'know' life! In this strange, terrible and ironic way, the living of life comes second to an unconscious and inexorable march towards its termination, with the lust for meaning fuelling the process. (Conversely and more positively, the relationship between life and death might be reflected, for those who can achieve it, in a conception of death and mortality that lends life greater depth and value).

While most of us would, of course, distance ourselves from such a grim-sounding and extreme position, I feel that this paradox dilutes itself to percolate into a state of conflict that we call 'human nature', and we create myths, stories and systems of belief because the paradox is almost too much to bear on its own. For most, transcendence is too much of an abstraction without such things. However, such conflict, human nature itself, is capable of extraordinary transmutation in the form of creativity and compassion and it is the assertion of this aspect of the human condition and the human propensity for hope, even in the most unimaginable circumstances, that provides inspiration and generates humanity itself.

In solving this tussle we do not simply face a choice between myth/faith and reductionism/pragmatism, though sometimes human beings seem to be polarised on such a spectrum. As already stated, *mythos* and *logos* have not always been considered mutually exclusive alternatives. Transcendence is a third 'way' if not exactly a 'middle way'. What's more, it doesn't invalidate the other two, connecting with both science and religious faith through the spirit of consciousness via metaphor.

Gary Zukav (1979) in *The Dancing Wu Li Masters* eloquently expresses the resonances of modern science and eastern mystical traditions and describes how these two planks of humanity converge, quoting physicist David Finkelstein thus:

> '. . . *a language of mythos, a language which alludes to experience but does not attempt to replace it or to mold our perception of it is the true language of physics. This is because not only the language that we use to communicate our daily experience, but also mathematics, follows a certain set of rules (classical logic). Experience itself is not bound by these rules. Experience follows a much more permissive set of rules (quantum logic). Quantum logic is not only more exciting than classical logic, it is more real. It is based not on the way we* think *of things, but upon the way we* experience *them.'*

Central theme

One of the central themes of this book is also cloaked in paradox. It is the apparent contradiction at the heart of good practitionership where the surrender of 'ego' and the humility that speaks of the highest state of *not knowing* (see previous chapter) couple with an all-important subjectivity through which the practitioner forges a personalised and informed connection with the patient in a unique bond or 'dance'. As practitioners, we learn, through both training and experience, a model, much data and many skills, such that we approach the patient positively primed with knowledge, understanding and ability. Yet, faced with the challenge of diagnosis and the technical demands of treatment, we do best when, having moved effectively and repeatedly between 'analysis' and 'synthesis' of the material, we come to that 'absence of ratiocination' as Tom Dummer would call it; that 'still', ego-less state which I've been at pains to extol. It is a state simultaneously full and 'void' as if, in the manner of a prism, we absorb the full, changing, kaleidoscopic spectrum and colour of knowledge, and through our 'art', produce a light that in its whiteness, purity and simplicity, is loaded with power; the power that makes therapeutic *entrainment* possible. Such a healing 'state' is a state of non-judgement, of 'ignorance' in its literal sense. Recalling Meister Eckhart, in order to achieve what he refers to as 'the interior act', we experience

> '*transformed knowledge; not ignorance which comes from lack of knowing; it is by knowing that we get to this unknowing . . .. We must sink into oblivion and ignorance. In this silence, this quiet, the Word is heard. There is no better method of approaching this Word than in silence, in quiet: we hear it and know it aright in unknowing.*'
>
> (Parke, 2009)

Some may have to forgive the implied parallels between the healing and spiritual modes that I have frequently insinuated in these chapters. But, as Zukav suggests, there *is* a growing sense of convergence between science (at the quantum end) and 'spirit', such that the practitioner state which I have attempted to describe, and that affords a truly holistic resonance with the patient's physical and energetic pattern in both diagnosis and treatment, seems closer and closer to that 'stillness' of which Eckhart, Heidegger and others speak. Eckhart again: '*you must draw all your powers to a point of stillness if you truly desire to experience the birth of God within yourself*' (Parke, 2009). It is not necessary to be a believer or to have any conscious 'spiritual' inclinations to hone one's skills in this way, or to take this statement too literally, but you might . . . Above all, this perspective is aspirational, not pretentious.

When William Sutherland borrowed the phrase 'be still and know' (Psalm 46:10), he helped refine a notion so valuable to osteopathic thought and practice. It contains the powerful reverential humility that underscores 'best practice'; but more than that, it insinuates the remarkable palpatory and conscious connection with the patient's 'pattern' that is achievable through the state of 'stillness' that I have tried to emphasise in this book; our very own example of paradox in action. In it, the mind stills to emptiness but is full of 'knowing'. Though still, it is active, searching, and its 'potency' is able to resonate and connect with the potency at the heart of the 'total lesion'.

It is probably true to say that the best treatments are always more than we can know, both in terms of what the patient 'does' with them and in terms of what they contain. Just as transcendence towards some kind of 'knowing' only follows its opposite, that is the doubt, surrender and acceptance of the fact that we cannot 'know', so healing treatments – however technically clothed – involve a 'submission' that follows knowledge, understanding and compassion, to allow for a resonance or entrainment to do their work. As I've said, Tom Dummer used to speak of the 'absence of ratiocination' at the moment of correction that followed a full resonance with the 'lesion' and its significance for the patient. When the stillness contained in the potency at the very heart of the patient's pattern can meet the stillness engendered by the practitioner in this way, the lesion is acknowledged or 'met' and the practitioner's grasp of the patient's 'next step' can begin. The technique of 'correction' enfolds this quality and gives expression to it and surely contains much of Eckhart's 'unknowing ignorance'.

CONCLUSION

To conclude, the thrill of validation through science, whilst putting flesh on the osteopathic bones of our art, does not really provide us with method, even if it energises it. The recent work on 'mechanotransduction' and the cytoskeleton is truly exciting. It is 21st century 'structure-and-function', but it is probably notionally what osteopaths have always known, even though we have had immense problems defining it. Our principles and contemporary science can be married in a union that will inspire us as osteopaths, though, as exciting as that is, it will not replace the process of synthesis that occurs uniquely in the relationship of each patient–practitioner exchange, that blending of consciousness that is fostered by the heart and humanity of the physician at his or her best. However, it is in the stillness of the therapeutic moment that we come close to one way of grasping the ungraspable: the wholeness that makes us all part of a resonating totality. It is something exquisite and 'true', but like all truth, the closer you approach it, the more it loses definition.

Perhaps the special beauty of analytical thought is glimpsed not when it achieves its goal – the moment of explanation – but when it doesn't; when it 'runs out of steam', out of words, and a mysterious void is reached that throws us back on to ourselves and the moment we experience. However, in that moment, perhaps, we inhabit the 'space', the inconceivable interval between particle and wave, or Heisenberg's strange kind of physical reality just in the middle between possibility and reality (Heisenberg, 1958). It is a moment that is neither ascent nor decline, as T.S Eliot put it in his *Four Quartets* (1944):

At the still point of the turning world. Neither flesh nor fleshless;
Neither from nor towards; at the still point, there the dance is,
But neither arrest nor movement. And do not call it fixity,
Where past and future are gathered. Neither movement from nor towards,
Neither ascent nor decline. Except for the point, the still point,
There would be no dance, and there is only the dance.

In that moment that couples an almost 'divine agnosticism' with the unique 'dance' with the patient's process, we contact its dynamic force and yoke it to something very uncertain indeed; a field of conscious potential perhaps. It is a process of total identification, harnessed to the most uncertain thing we know, maybe Aristotle's 'plenum', or the zero point field, that mysterious 'void' or energetic 'soup' that we all inhabit. And we do it via an intelligent, knowing 'fulcrum', and that strange but profound quality of stillness; and in that fusion, healing occurs. Perhaps 'miracle' always resides at the heart of paradox.

REFERENCES

Eliot, T S, 1944, *Four Quartets*, Faber and Faber.
Heisenberg, W, 1958, *Physics and Philosophy*, Harper Torch Books.
Parke, S, 2009, *Conversations with Meister Eckhart*, White Crow Books.
Watts, A, 1951, *The Wisdom of Insecurity*, Pantheon Books.
Zukav, G, 1979, *The Dancing Wu Li Masters*, Hutchinson.

Chapter 15

Epilogue – tying it together: spirit, humanity and the art of practice

> Observing the relationship between science and art, Raymond Chandler once said: *'There are two kinds of truth; the truth that lights the way and the truth that warms the heart'*
>
> **(Chandler, 1976).**

How does our science link with the spirit and humanity in the work to produce the art of practice? And just how does knowledge distil itself into the synthesis that *is* the moment of treatment?

Some might struggle, with some justification, to see the relevance of the foregoing philosophical musings to the practice of any therapeutic discipline or, more particularly, to the practice of osteopathy; that armed with a reasonable grasp of concepts, theories, medical science and therapeutic methods, we should be adequately equipped to have a stab at the measures required to resuscitate health in our patients or, at least, make them more comfortable. With all this knowledge and ability, we should have the ingredients to put the recipe together without all that flabby philosophy.

And speaking of recipes, many cooks tell of the frustration of attempting to emulate the creation of a fine chef, only to find that it doesn't quite come off; some crucial ingredient lacking! Many will even say that the dish only 'works' if prepared and cooked 'with love'. My mentor, Tom Dummer, was one such cook! The problem, if it is a problem, with the 'osteopathic practitioner recipe' is that osteopathy is a concept and only 'exists' in reality *as* it is being practised. The 'human' ingredient in all its complexity is the only thing that energises all other ingredients; so that the psychological, experiential, empathic and technical qualities in the practitioner coalesce uniquely to permit access to, and interpretation of, the patient's 'material', itself an expression of *their* humanity.

As I've said many times in this book, rationality has its limits. Skills do not develop through greater knowledge but through the *application* and *processing* of knowledge; a process that sees the exponent occupy a position that is 'enmeshed in the detail', in the spaces between the elements of knowledge and understanding. It is because our work is concerned with an individuated or highly personalised context in which the clinical problem is biomechanically and bioenergetically enfolded, that the intangible elements of 'function' are found to be inseparably entwined with what is rationally 'available' or accessible to us. When we engage and touch the patient, we hold a world of being whose elements sustain the complex patterning of each individual that expresses health as well as its opposite. Any holistic method ignores these subtleties at its peril and therefore has to create a model that can encompass them.

In the end, the art of osteopathy resides in the facility to resonate with the 'total lesion' in order to read, acknowledge, understand and relate to it. Such a facility is generated by a perspective and attitude that are partly about a means of moving back and forth in our minds between the analysis of detail and the creation, through an 'orchestrated' synthesis, of a working 'pattern' based on osteopathic principles. This mental fluctuation is married to a 'stillness' and a humility that are born of 'doubt' – one might almost say 'wonder' – in the sense that doubt is the opposite of dogma. And by this I mean an openness to what *is* rather than a rational sense of certainty or of analytical detail *on its own*. Recalling Meister Eckhart once more (Parke 2009), remember that we arrive at this position *after* the assimilation of fact and detail (viewed, for us, through our 'osteopathic lens'). In a culture based on the need and the quest for certainty, this may seem counter-intuitive. But it is this position that enables us to join the 'dance' and to find the stillness from which to work so that an 'entrainment' can occur along with the liberation of the healing potential within each patient. This humility is not some precious credo; it is the place from which the 'view' is unquestionably clearer and the connection with the patient's clinical detail more 'true'. This is conceptually and procedurally at odds with so much within the conventional scientific and medical paradigms; it is no wonder that impenetrable barriers have endured.

THAT 'STILL LEVERAGE FULCRUM'

This crucial position of 'doubt' involves an attitude that allows for the idea of *possibility beyond what can be fully and explicitly known,* and of moving beyond 'ego', even though this might at first seem to contradict the importance of the 'subjective' that I have wished to emphasise. But it is my view that such 'doubt', such uncertainty, engender an attitude that is 'clear', 'non-judgemental' and profoundly 'still'; perhaps Heidegger's *listening, receptive attitude* (Heidegger, 1976). It is a state both pregnant with knowledge and skill whilst at the same moment being a state of perceptive, psychological, intellectual, tactile, even ethical *neutrality* that begins simply (in training at least) as a state of physical 'inertia' and receptivity; a process or technique we teach in some approaches as the use of the *fulcrum,* a 'still leverage' point that we create in our palpating touch. (It often involves the use of the forearms or elbows – virtually 'liberating' the hands to 'move' or resonate with the motile patterns within the patient's tissues – but, in truth, it can be anywhere. Later, it becomes less 'physical' and more a matter of perceptual orientation, the stillness becoming established in the practitioner in the form of an 'attitude'.) Quantum theory supports this almost philosophical position in its emphasis on our 'role' in a participatory world that is always incompletely and imperfectly 'known' to our observational faculties. Against this background, the 'still, listening fulcrum' allows for a deeper contact and resonance with the patient's 'real' lesion process, that pattern of dysfunction that we, as osteopaths, connect with the patient's presenting state or condition.

So the process that follows the assimilation of fact and detail gives us a vocabulary; our model gives us the grammar; we fashion the ability to refine and 'speak' the language with fluency, but it is the stillness that creates the poetry out of it all. And where mind, body and spirit coalesce or conjoin, it is only 'poetry' that will do. This, as in any discipline, is where the potential for the 'art' of good practice resides.

Searching questions

So much of what we do is based on the knowledge and visualisation of anatomy and a conceptual link with its significance in any particular case. As we alight upon areas of dysfunction that we evaluate in regard to the parameters we've looked at, we 'ask' many questions including the following:

- What is the nature of the disturbance?
- What is its potential significance anatomically and physiologically?
- What are its relationships with the rest of the structure and other somatic dysfunctions? In other words, what is its global or 'whole-body' significance?
- How are such interactions likely to reflect the patient's history?
- How are they likely to reflect the symptomatology?
- What is the significance of our findings in terms of pathology?
- What are the psycho-emotional ramifications if any?
- How are these findings 'patterned' according to osteopathic principles (structure/function 'bonds')?
- Does this pattern express a dominant 'theme', e.g. torsion, transverse or lateral strain, compression, intersegmental dysfunction, 'positional' lesion, kyphoscoliosis or other dominant quality? Is it 'articular', soft tissue, fascial, 'energetic', etc.?

- Can the *stillness* in the observational and palpatory process refine our diagnostic assessment so far?
- Does the pattern contain an identifiable focus; is it 'accessible'/treatable; what is its quality or flavour?
- Is the patient able to sustain and respond to the treatment envisaged, and is it safe?

And remarkably, the answers to these questions are rapidly integrated in the practitioner's assessment of the patient in that moment to form a resonant connection with the patient's tissues and process that 'melts' into treatment.

It is the extraordinary way that these diagnostic elements fuse into a single notion that guide our work with the patient and that probably underlie those early remarks to students at the beginning of the lecture series I gave at the ESO for many years, along the lines that I couldn't really show them how to *do* osteopathy (as opposed to technique). I used to draw three interlocking or overlapping circles; one circle would represent the patient and all their interwoven 'material' (history, trauma, personality, predispositions, symptoms, etc.). The second circle would represent the many osteopathic constructs and their interplay (as discussed earlier in this book). And the third represented the practitioner, their skills, understanding, attitude, technical orientation, power of empathy etc. I'd then shade the area of overlap and, in one of my early flights into abstraction, claim that my aim was to help them 'get into that particular place of overlap'; a place in which the synthesis of the patient's data, sieved through the conceptual osteopathic 'mesh' is yoked to the empathic, resonant skills, perception and understanding of the practitioner, rather in the manner of Zen, to engender what we'd later refer to as the *entrainment* of a *coherent* pattern. This is the 'point of stillness' that permits the work to go beyond mere technique, to access the healing moments in the patient through their own therapeutic 'still points', those moments in which the gathering of the vast potential for healing allow real change to occur. (Such 'still points' are variously conceived relating sometimes to a stilling of the potency in the fluctuant fluids of the body with a resultant recalibration of biochemical, neural and bioelectrical information; and sometimes echoing the effects of the 'still leverage fulcrum' that the practitioner uses to read and access the patient's 'mechanism').

Aside from Heisenberg's uncertainty principle, I sometimes wonder whether quantum theory has left us with a view of the significance of 'uncertainty' in general, along with a randomness in our world so different from the Newtonian ideal. Perhaps life with its unfathomable seamless wholeness – to some, an almost theistic notion – is represented by the 'wave function' of energy or matter, with its 'home' in another mystery called *consciousness*. To try to understand it in its entirety is futile as the process of observation will

always 'collapse the wave' and we are left with decontextualised approxima-
tions. After all, how can consciousness appraise itself? It is as if we are only
able to get *so* near, so that life's experience has to be 'lived' rather than 'known'.

To accept the limitation of analytical thought is to place a value on experience – subjective experience – that is at least equal in importance to knowledge. It then remains a matter of opinion as to whether this position is
acceptable for the proper practice of healing and medicine. If it is, then there
is a part of it that will always be an art. And as the biological sciences reveal
more and more of the complex interacting biorhythmic oscillations that create
'coherence' in health, the sum of those parts will probably always remain
slightly out of reach in our attempts to define *life*. Its secrets will, I feel, remain
enfolded in the same domain as the 'art' of healing, despite all our efforts to
define its ingredients and teach its skills to others.

In all probability, we will learn more and more about the mechanism by
which the practitioner engages the patient's 'field', resonates with it, even
entrains it; but ultimately the process will still be based on the way one human
being *engages* another and how the 'dance' is driven by human qualities,
values and instincts. Just *where* and *how* these qualities coalesce will probably
remain a mystery, a thing of wonder. As ever, method and technique are mere
vehicles for a complex process underpinned by knowledge, empathy and
resonance that are part of the 'dance' of human interaction and creativity –
one modulated by a special set of expectations, demands and intentions.

Long before my acquaintance with the delightful lecturer of my opening
remarks, my grandmother would put 'learning' in its place by opining – with
hundreds of other grandmothers, no doubt – that 'it's not *what* you know, it's
who you know' that helps you get on in the world. In teaching students over
the years, I found myself repeating the phrase: 'it's not so much what you
know as *who you are*' that helps to define good practice.

So much of the foregoing is just one person's journey through the mire of
knowing *and* being, or more accurately, the on-going process of learning and
becoming, and the way that they shape a reasonable attempt at practice. For
in the end, unless we go beyond 'scientism' in the practice of (osteopathic)
medicine and temper our knowledge, insight, understanding and method
with humanity, we fall short in the process of earning the trust of those we
purport to help. *They* are the focus of our endeavours rather than the rigours
of science or even the art of osteopathy itself.

And as we contemplate the unknowable and whether the greatest creative
achievements of Mozart or Beethoven or Shakespeare are proof of a god or
not, we could perhaps arrive at a place where we might instead deepen our
definition or conception of God to reach a complete abstraction, one that
engenders wonder rather than reverence.

So, to end, I'd like to leave you something from Alan Watts' *The Wisdom of Insecurity* (1951) that says so much about what, for most of us, is so hard to articulate but which I feel might have meaning for everyone: practitioners, patients or anyone at all.

'The more [the scientist] analyses the universe into infinitesimals, the more things he finds to classify, and the more he perceives the relativity of all classification. What he does not know seems to increase in geometric progression to what he knows. Steadily he approaches the point where what is unknown is not a mere blank space in the web of words but a window in the mind, a window whose name is not ignorance but wonder.

*The timid mind shuts this window with a bang, and is silent and thoughtless about what it does not know, in order to chatter the more about what it thinks it knows. It fills up the uncharted spaces with mere repetition of what has always been explored. But the open mind knows that the most minutely explored territories have not really been known at all, but only marked and measured a thousand times over. And the fascinating mystery of what it is that we mark and measure must in the end "tease us out of thought" until the mind forgets to circle and to pursue its own processes, and becomes aware that **to be** at this moment is pure miracle.'*

REFERENCES

Chandler, R, 1976, *The Notebooks of Raymond Chandler*, reprinted 2007, Harper Perennial.
Heidegger, M, 1976, Only a god can save us, *Der Speigel* (vol 30, no 23).
Parke, S, 2009, *Conversations with Meister Eckhart*, White Crow Books.
Watts, A, 1951, *The Wisdom of Insecurity*, Pantheon Books.

Bibliography

Armstrong, Karen, 2009, *The Case for God*, The Bodley Head.

Becker, Rollin, 1997, *Life in Motion*, Rudra Press.

Brooks, Michael, 2010, *Thirteen Things That Don't Make Sense*, Profile Books.

Capra, Ftitjof, 1975, *The Tao of Physics*, Fontana.

Chown, Marcus, 2006, *Quantum Theory Cannot Hurt You: A Guide to the Universe*, Faber and Faber.

Dossey, Larry, 1982, *Space, Time and Medicine*, Shambhala Publications.

Eliot, T S, 1944, *Four Quartets*, Faber and Faber.

Feynman, Richard, 1988, *What Do You Care What Other People Think?* Norton & Co.

Frankl, Vicktor, 1946, *Man's Search for Meaning*, Beacon Press.

Fulford, Robert, ed Cisler, Theresa, 2003, *Are We On The Path?* The Cranial Academy.

Goswami, Amit, 1993, *The Self-Aware Universe*, Putnam Penguin (1995).

Gray, John, 2002, *Straw Dogs*, Granta Books.

Gray, John, 2011, *The Immortality Commission*, Allen Lane.

Handoll, Nicholas, 2000, *The Anatomy of Potency*, Osteophathic Supplies Ltd.

Helman, Cecil, 1991, *Body Myths*, Chatto & Windus.

Herbert, Nick, 1985, *Quantum Reality*, Anchor Books.

Herbert, Nick, 1993, *Elemental Mind*, Dutton.

Ho, Mae-Wan, 2008, *The Rainbow and the Worm*, World Scientific Publishing.

Ingber, Donald, 2008, Tensegrity and mechanotransduction, *Journal of Bodywork and Movement Therapies* 12:198–200.

Korr, Irvin, 1979, *The Collected Papers of Irvin Korr*, American Academy of Osteopathy.

Korr, Irvin, 1967, *The Physiological Basis of Osteopathic Medicine*, The Postgraduate Institute of Osteopathic Medicine and Surgery.

Korr, Irvin, 1977, *The Neurobiologic Mechanisms in Manipulative Therapy*, Plenum.

Lee, R Paul, 2005, *Interface: Mechanisms of Spirit in Osteopathy*, Stillness Press.

Lever, Robert, 1981, An osteopathic orientation within a social context, *Journal of the Society of Osteopaths* 10:9–13.

Lipton, Bruce, 2005, *The Biology of Belief*, Hay House.

Lorimer, David, 1998, *The Spirit of Science*, The Wrekin Trust.

McTaggart, Lynne, 2001, *The Field*, Harper Collins.

Oschman, James, 2000, *Energy Medicine*, Churchill Livingstone.

Oschman, James, 2003, *Energy Medicine in Therapeutics and Human Performance*, Butterworth-Heinemann.

Parke, Simon, 2009, *Conversations with Meister Eckhart*, White Crow Books.

Parsons, John & Marcer, Nicholas, 2006, *Osteopathy*, Churchill Livingstone.

Peat, F David, 2007, *Pathways of Chance*, Pari Publishing.

Pert, Candace, 1997, *The Molecules of Emotion*, Simon & Schuster.

Pischinger, Alfred, 2007, *The Extracellular Matrix and Ground Regulation*, North Atlantic Books.

Sacks, Oliver, 1984, *A Leg to Stand On*, Picador.

Smith, Fritz, 1998, *Inner Bridges*, Humanics New Age.

Still, Andrew, 1892, *Philosophy and Mechanical Principles of Osteopathy*, repub. 1986, Osteopathic Enterprise.

Sutherland, William, ed Wales, Anne, 1990, *Teachings in the Science of Osteopathy*, Sutherland Cranial Teaching Foundation.

Sutherland, William, 1967, *Contributions of Thought*, Sutherland Cranial Teaching Foundation.

Watts, Alan, 1936, *The Spirit of Zen*, John Murray.

Watts, Alan, 1951, *The Wisdom of Insecurity*, Pantheon Books.

Zukav, Gary, 1979, *The Dancing Wu Li Masters*, Hutchinson.

Index